MICROSCOPY HANDBOOKS 46

Image Cytometry

Royal Microscopical Society MICROSCOPY HANDBOOKS

Series Advisors

Angela Köhler (Life Sciences), *Alfred Wegener Institut, Notke-Strasse 85, 22607 Hamburg, Germany*

Mark Rainforth (Materials Sciences), *Department of Engineering Materials, University of Sheffield, Sheffield S1 3JD, UK*

Image Cytometry

P. Chieco[a], A. Jonker[b] and C.J.F. van Noorden[b]
[a]Institute of Oncology "Felice Addarii", Bologna, Italy,
[b]Department of Cell Biology and Histology, Academic
Medical Center, University of Amsterdam, The Netherlands

In association with the Royal Microscopical Society

A CIP catalogue record for this book is available from the British Library.

ISBN 1 85996 173 8

BIOS Scientific Publishers Ltd
9 Newtec Place, Magdalen Road, Oxford OX4 1RE, UK
Tel. +44 (0)1865 726286. Fax +44 (0)1865 246823
World Wide Web home page: http://www/bios.co.uk/

Published in the United States of America, its dependent territories and Canada by Springer-Verlag New York Inc., 175 Fifth Avenue, New York, NY 10010-7858, in association with BIOS Scientific Publishers Ltd.

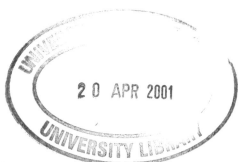

Production Editor: Paul Barlass
Typeset by Marksbury Multimedia Ltd, Midsomer Norton, Bath, UK
Printed by Biddles Ltd., Guildford, UK, www.biddles.co.uk

Front cover: The images illustrate three typical preparations suitable for image analysis. The underlying image (top left, bottom right) shows a routine cytological specimen where isolated cells can easily be measured. The top right image shows a stereological counting frame and a grid overlaying a histological section to quantify immunological-labeled cells. The bottom left image shows a gray level histogram overlaid on a liver tissue section.

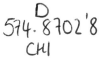

Contents

Abbreviations

A/D	analog to digital
AGC	automatic gain control
APS	active pixel sensor
AU	arbitrary units
BMP	bit-mapped format
CCD	charge coupled device
CCIR	Comité Consultatif International des Radio Communications
CCTV	closed-circuit TV
CID	charge injection device
CMOS	complementary metal oxide semiconductors
DA	disk apertures
DMA	direct memory access
DNL	difference nonlinearity
DSP	digital signal processing
EIA	Electronics Industry Association
FITC	fluorescein isothiocyanate
FOV	field of view
FRP	final reaction product
GL	gray level
IOD	integral optical density
JPEG	joint photographic expert group
λ	wavelength
LED	light-emitting diode
LI	labeling index
LSB	least significant bit
LUT	look-up table
MOS	metal oxide semiconductors
MPEG	moving picture expert group
NA	numerical aperture
NE	electrons produced by dark current
NP	electrons produced by pre-amplifier noise
NTSC	National Television Systems Committee
NT	total noise
OD	optical density
PAL	phase-alternating line system
PCI	peripheral component interconnect
PLL	phase locked loop

RAM	random access memory
RGB	red, green and blue
S/N	signal-to-noise
SD	standard deviation
SDK	software development kit
T	transmission
TDI	time delay and integration
TIFF	tagged image file format
TRITC	tetramethylrhodamine isothiocyanate
UMA	unified memory architecture

Preface

This guide is intended as a simple, yet detailed, compendium of the technical principles of image cytometry. It also includes practical descriptions of operative protocols and benchmark procedures. Tips are regularly provided to solve problems and avoid errors. The book bridges the technological gap between the complex studies performed up to the 1980s, which established the principles of quantitative microscopy, and modern computerized cytometric methods using solid state cameras. Thus, the basic cytometric techniques and principles are all covered in terms of image cytometry. Key theories and procedures are concisely set out. The book has been written to help scientists correctly apply quantitative microscopical imaging of cells and tissues with a minimum of fuss.

P. Chieco, A. Jonker, C.J.F. Van Noorden

Acknowledgements

We would like to acknowledge Gabriele Vanni, D. Eng. (electronic) for his assistance in writing chapters related to cameras and hardware; Mr Robin MT Cooke helping us make the text as reader friendly as possible; and Mr Jan Peeterse for helping in the preparation of the figures.

To Edward S. Reynolds, MD

1 Introduction

This book provides a brief guide to 'image cytometry', a powerful quantitative tool based on microscopy and digital imaging. Image cytometry may be considered as a particular sector of scientific imaging, a field that also includes video microscopy, image analysis and image processing. Cytometry is about obtaining correct measurements in cells and tissues. Essentially, measurements that interest are either planar (areas, lengths, profiles, etc.) or photometric (absorbance and fluorescence measurement and luminometry). Therefore, cytometry relies on careful calibration and control of acquisition of digital images that are stored in a computer memory and evaluated with image analysis programs. The software used for cytometry may either take the form of general image analysis software or may be designed for a specific purpose. In either case, it has to be capable of assisting cytometrists in the fundamental requirements of their work: calibration, interactivity, speed and sampling. This book will deal with all of these aspects.

As cytometry is a measuring technique, the need for instrument calibration is obvious. On the other hand, general experts in image analysis may not always be aware that easy interactivity with the software is a particular requirement in cytometry. Indeed, modern system analysts prefer to emphasize the more or less complete automation of their software in image processing and analysis. Sophisticated automation is rarely useful in cytometry. Our daily experience has taught us that it is much easier to select objects interactively than to waste time correcting errors introduced in images processed by automatic algorithms. The need for easy interactivity with the software is due to the wide variety of objects that have to be measured and the fact that automatic image algorithms are incapable of identifying them appropriately. A light microscopical object may be constituted of either isolated cultured cells that can be easily segmented by automatic procedures, or of tissue sections or cytological preparations where automation does not work. Think for instance of situations where we need to measure structures that require identification by an experienced microscopist: areas of normal epithelium, dysplasia and differentiated or undifferentiated cancer in a biopsy; different cell types in a kidney glomerulus; different layers of cells in an epithelium, and so on. Even in electron microscopy, with the fine differences in gray levels that distinguish subcellular structures, or in phase contrast microscopy, with its high light scattering, automation does not work at all well. There are a number of situations where a stereological grid super-imposed on the image works far better and faster than sophisticated segmentation algorithms. For this reason, cytometry software needs to provide a variety of tools that allow one to select interactively the most appropriate strategy for measurement.

Closely linked with the interactivity problem is the speed of analysis. In cytometry, we analyze populations of objects and frequently we want to detect heterogeneity within the populations. For each specimen, we have to collect tens or hundreds of objects and we often have to make more than one measurement per object. For example, we may need to measure telomere length of human chromosomes (46 chromosomes per cell with two telomeres each) in a heterogeneous cell population (Poon *et al.*, 1999). For this reason, cytometric software and hardware have to be able to produce rapid measurements. The 'do more less well' principle applied in stereology and cancer screening translates as 'do more less complex' in cytometry, meaning that we have to perform simple measurements in an object sample that is as representative as possible (Gundersen and Osterby, 1980).

As cytometry deals with populations of objects, unbiased sampling procedures are of paramount importance. The final analysis of our specimen usually does not result in a single number, but in a series of values, from which means, standard deviations, counts or frequency histograms are derived. To be representative for a particular specimen, measurements must be taken with a comprehensive randomization scheme at all levels.

Image cytometry was originally known either as plain 'cytometry', or as 'cytophotometry'. Cytometry stemmed from the need to quantify substances in cells. It came into existence in the thirties when the first attempt was made to quantify amounts of unstained DNA in nuclei by means of absorbances of ultraviolet light (Caspersson, 1936), and then branched out during the following decades. The transformation of microscopes into 'microphoto(fluoro)meters' enabled various cellular components and enzymatic activities to be quantified by measuring light emitted or absorbed by stained or unstained cells or tissue sections (Altman, 1975; Caspersson and Kudynowski, 1980; Pattison et al., 1979; Piller, 1977). However, microphotometers are much more complex than photometers, and measuring in cells is not the same thing as measuring solutions in a cuvette. It soon became clear that just using monochro-matic light and attaching a photometric head to an ocular was not sufficient for valid cytometry. So, in the period between 1940 and 1980 a great deal of work was performed to understand the principles of microscope photometry and to avoid serious measuring errors caused by factors such as scattered or stray light, chromatic aberrations, and the lack of uniformity of stained objects (Goldstein, 1970, 1971, 1981; Ornstein, 1952; Van Noorden and Butcher, 1986). In the first half of the

1980s, the most advanced microscope photometers were based on the principle of raster scanning: objects were rapidly scanned by a thin cone of monochromatic light (0.2–0.5 μm in diameter in the plane of the specimen). After being scanned in this way, each object was represented by an array of tens or hundreds of optical density (OD) values in the *x–y* dimension (*Figure 1.1*). The size and the integrated and mean ODs of an object could be determined by setting a threshold and summing up all the ODs. Scanning with a small measuring spot was the most widely adopted procedure to reconstruct the planar form of objects and to perform correct photometric measurements (Altman, 1975). Indeed, dyes and stained molecules in cells are so heterogeneously distributed that it is necessary to divide the object in a very large number of tiny measurement spots. In this way, we can be reasonably sure that the dye distribution in each measurement spots is homogeneous, and thus reasonably similar to the clear solution in a photometric cuvette (Goldstein, 1971; Ornstein, 1952).

To gain a better idea of how image cytometry was so revolutionary in this field, it is interesting to consider the main drawbacks of microscope photometers:

(i) The scanning of the object under the microscope was obtained with rapid and regular movements of the light source (flying spot) or the microscope stage (scanning stage) (Altman, 1975). The illuminating diaphragm had to be just slightly larger than the measuring spot in order to eliminate the stray light and this requirement created serious problems related to the correct alignment and focusing of the optics (Goldstein, 1970). Cytophotometers were therefore complex and expensive instruments that were accessible only to dedicated research laboratories. They had to be operated by highly trained specialists, usually at the Ph.D. level.

(ii) To reduce the dimensions of the measurement spot to a diameter of 0.2–0.5 μm, high-power immersion objectives with a very narrow depth of field had to be used. This introduced focusing errors when the entire thickness of the object was not in focus in a single plane.

Figure 1.1. Schematic drawing of a cell with a stained nucleus (gray) rasterized by a scanning spot. Scanning microphotometers collect only numbers and do not display the image of the cell on a monitor. To determine the area and thus the mean absorbance of the nucleus, it is necessary to examine the frequency histogram of OD values and set a threshold that excludes the low values corresponding to the cell cytoplasm and extracellular surrounding.

```
0.05 0.08 0.01 0.02 0.08 0.07 0.02 0.08 0.04 0.01
0.05 0.02 0.08 0.07 0.01 0.02 0.07 0.06 0.07 0.03
0.02 0.04 0.08 0.05 0.08 0.07 0.04 0.06 0.04 0.07
0.07 0.08 0.02 0.07 0.06 0.04 0.05 0.08 0.01 0.04
0.04 0.05 0.04 0.09 0.27 0.09 0.02 0.05 0.01 0.03
0.08 0.03 0.65 0.57 0.91 0.96 0.77 0.03 0.05 0.03
0.05 0.09 0.7  1.42 1.19 1.29 0.63 0.02 0.01 0.01
0.04 0.07 0.72 0.93 1.53 1.38 0.8  0.01 0.05 0.04
0.02 0.10 1.08 1.55 1.23 1.36 1.14 0.48 0.03 0.08
0.01 0.05 1.16 1.16 1.13 1.05 1.1  0.68 0.07 0.01
0.08 0.05 1.17 1.17 1.51 0.96 0.97 0.72 0.06 0.01
0.05 0.02 1.2  1.28 0.95 1.26 1.19 0.69 0.04 0.05
0.02 0.06 1.12 1.11 1.39 1.39 0.8  0.6  0.03 0.03
0.04 0.06 0.84 1.38 1.57 1.52 1.09 0.62 0.01 0.04
0.05 0.07 0.91 1.59 1.34 1.36 1.15 0.52 0.03 0.03
0.02 0.05 1    1.29 1.00 1.33 1.01 0.14 0.07 0.01
0.04 0.03 0.78 0.95 1.38 1.13 0.72 0.05 0.07 0.04
0.02 0.08 0.74 1.36 1.38 0.98 0.58 0.03 0.04 0.08
0.03 0.08 0.58 0.53 0.76 0.57 0.56 0.04 0.07 0.06
0.07 0.02 0.04 0.09 0.02 0.03 0.10 0.02 0.07 0.03
0.07 0.07 0.09 0.10 0.03 0.06 0.08 0.05 0.02 0.05
0.03 0.08 0.02 0.03 0.07 0.06 0.04 0.02 0.02 0.02
0.08 0.03 0.03 0.06 0.06 0.07 0.03 0.03 0.07 0.03
0.05 0.01 0.03 0.02 0.04 0.04 0.01 0.01 0.05 0.04
```

(iii) Scanning cytophotometers were not suitable for measuring tissue structures larger than single nuclei or cells, or at most groups of cells in a tissue section.

(iv) Although cytofluorometric measurements that involved quantification of light emitted by dyes bound to cell structures were less demanding and could be made with larger measuring spots (2–20 µm of diameter), scanning cytophotometers were not easily adaptable to fluorometry, particularly because of fluorescence decay, quenching and fading.

Things changed radically in the second half of the 1980s with the arrival of solid-state cameras and the increasing availability of cheap computers. Modern instrumentation for image cytometry is much more reliable and easier to operate than the most expensive cytophotometer of the early eighties. All the new developments were based on solid-state sensors of the charge coupled device (CCD) type, which were now being mounted on consumer, industrial or scientific video cameras. CCD sensors collect images from the object and transmit them to a computer. The sensors are small silicon chips made up of thousands of tiny square or rectangular photoelements arranged in an array of lines and columns (Aikens, 1990). Each photoelement, a few microns wide, collects photons from the object and transforms them into electrons (known as photoelectrons) that are transmitted through a serial register and a video cable to the computer where the image can be reconstructed and displayed on a monitor. For a particular range of light intensities, each photoelement acts as a high-fidelity photometric unit, producing a signal that is proportional to the intensity of the incident light.

In the above context, the success of image cytometry was determined by a few key factors:

(i) The image becomes electronically scanned in thousands or millions of photometric spots without the need for any moving part in the instrumentation.

(ii) The size of the photoelements in the CCD camera is smaller than the smallest measuring spot of the scanning-stage or flying-spot microphotometers.

(iii) The small size of photoelements allows the use of objectives with a large depth of field, thereby reducing 'out-of-focus' problems. When using $40 \times$ or $20 \times$ objectives, a photoelement size of 8 µm in the CCD camera reduces a photometric spot to 0.2 and 0.4 µm, respectively, in the specimen plane. These sizes are sufficient to avoid distributional errors, and allow measurements to be made of large areas of the specimen (for example entire tissue sections).

(iv) The spectral response and the quantum efficiency of CCDs are satisfactory at all visible wavelengths. CCDs may also be used for infrared microscopy.

(v) The response to light of CCD chips is linear even at particularly short or long exposures. CCDs may integrate the incoming light for seconds or even minutes. This was not possible with thermionic tubes and photometric heads.

(vi) The possibility to visualize the image to be measured directly on the monitor greatly simplifies microscope adjustments.

(vii) Planar, stereological, fluorescence and absorbance measurements can all be carried out with the same instrument.

References

Aikens, R.S. (1990) CCD cameras for video microscopy. In: *Optical Microscopy for Biology* (eds B. Herman and K. Jacobson), Wiley-Liss, New York, pp. 207–218.

Altman, F.P. (1975) Quantitation in histochemistry: a review of some commercially available microdensitometers. *Histochem. J.* **7:** 375–395.

Caspersson, T. (1936) Über den chemischen Aufbau der Strukturen des Zellkernes. *Scand. Arch. Physiol.* **73:** Suppl 8.

Caspersson, T. and Kudynowski, J. (1980) Cytochemical instrumentation for cytopathological work. *Int. Rev. Exp. Pathol.* **21:** 1–54.

Goldstein, D.J. (1970) Aspects of scanning microdensitometry. I. Stray light (glare). *J. Microsc.* **92:** 1–16.

Goldstein, D.J. (1971) Aspects of scanning microdensitometry. II. Spot size, focus and resolution. *J. Microsc.* **93:** 15–42.

Goldstein, D.J. (1981) Errors in microdensitometry. *Histochem. J.* **13:** 251–267.

Gundersen, H.J.G. and Osterby, R. (1980) Optimizing sampling efficiency of stereological studies in biology: or 'Do more less well'. *J. Microsc.* **121:** 65–73.

Ornstein, L. (1952) The distributional error in microspectrophotometry. *Lab. Invest.* **1:** 250–262.

Pattison, J.R., Bitensky, L. and Chayen, J. (eds) (1979) *Quantitative Cytochemistry and its Applications.* Academic Press, London.

Piller, H. (1977) *Microscope Photometry.* Springer-Verlag, Berlin.

Poon, S.S.S., Martens, U.M., Ward, R.K. and Lansdorp, P.M. (1999) Telomere length measurements using digital fluorescence microscopy. *Cytometry* **36:** 267–278.

Van Noorden C.J.F. and Butcher R.G. (1986) The out-of-range error in microdensitometry. *Histochem. J.* **18:** 397–398.

2 Instrumentation

2.1 Image capturing

Image analysis systems may acquire images from video cameras, still cameras, video recorders and scanners. In microscopy, images are captured by a camera mounted on a microscope and transmitted to a computer through a digitizer or a framegrabber card. The framegrabber either sends the image to the computer random access memory (RAM) or to the computer monitor (*Figure 2.1*). The imager in a camera may be a thermionic tube (Vidicon, Chalnicon) or a solid-state sensor. Today, the imagers of choice for use in quantitative imaging systems are of the solid-state type, mostly CCD sensors. Other sensors used in cameras are

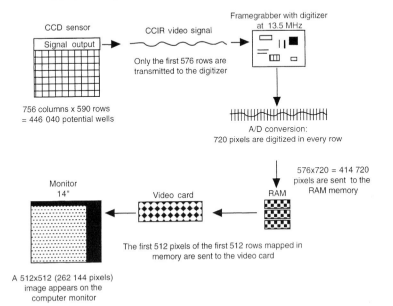

Figure 2.1. Drawing of the video signal trail in the image analysis system. This schematic figure shows how a 756×590 signal from a CCD sensor with rectangular pixels is transformed into a 512×512 image with square pixels.

charge injection devices (CID) or complementary metal oxide semiconductors (CMOS).

2.1.1 *Image sensors*

Charge coupled device sensors. Charge coupled device sensors (*Figure 2.2*), which were invented at Bell Laboratories in 1969 (Boyle and Smith, 1970), are silicon-based chips composed of a series of closely spaced columns (channels), each subdivided along its length by tiny independent photoelements parceling images in thousands or even millions of individual picture elements (pixels). Photoelements are tiny silicon cells that convert radiation into electric energy. Light falling on the photoelements is absorbed by the crystalline silicon, where it breaks bonds, displacing a number of electrons proportional to the amount of incident photons. A set of tiny polysilicon electrodes (also known as 'gates') positioned on the surface of each photoelement creates a buried electron depletion region (potential well) which collects the charges displaced from the silicon substrate (Kristian and Blouke, 1982). After a set time interval ranging from microseconds to seconds and even minutes, these packets of photoelectrons are transferred row by row to a serial register and then to an output amplifier where they are converted to a video signal representative for the optical image on the sensor. As the name suggests, the serial register is a one-dimensional horizontal row of cells that collects, row by row, the photoelectrons of the two-dimensional image area (known as the 'parallel register') and sends them in a 'serial' manner, pixel after pixel, row after row, to the output amplifier. The latter transforms each electrical charge packet into a voltage, reading out the entire row. The process is repeated until the entire image area has been read, thus providing a video signal. It is worth mentioning that although the video signal originates from a solid-state chip, the signal is actually 'analog' and needs to be converted into a digital signal after the output amplifier. Thus, the CCD sensor serves as an image collecting device, and is the first step in the signal transmission pathway.

To gain a working knowledge of CCDs, it is important to know that a CCD is actually a simple series connection of metal-oxide-semiconductor (MOS) capacitors and that the sensor itself behaves as a type of charge

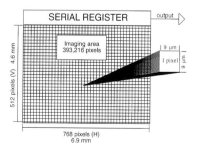

Figure 2.2. Scheme of a typical CCD sensor. The imaging area is formed by a parallel register of photoelements that moves the luminous signals row by row to the serial register. Reproduced from Aikens *et al* (1989) Solid-state imagers for microscopy. *Methods in Cell Biology* **16**: 291–313, with permission of Academic Press.

A CCD sensor is formed by thousands or millions of potential wells that behave as photoelements since they collect electrons originating from photons. These photoelements, which are commonly referred to as *pixels* (short for picture elements), are the smallest units in which images can be segmented.

storage and transport device (Theuwissen, 1995). The capacitor in each photoelement in the chip is a potential well, collecting the charges (electrons) originating from the photoelements. It is the user who establishes, by adjusting the electronic settings of the video camera, at what time intervals the charges are read by emptying the potential wells. For example, if the user establishes that a 483-row CCD sensor of a given video camera must emit a standard RS-170 video signal, each row (and, therefore, all the photoelements in that row) is read and emptied every 33 ms. Although practical potential well capacities reach as many as a million electrons (Aikens *et al.*, 1989), they will overflow into surrounding photoelements when the sensor is constantly illuminated and charges are not read out. This overflow is called blooming.

Blooming occurs in CCD sensors when photoelectrons in a potential well spill into surrounding potential wells. It happens when the well is strongly illuminated and the photoelements are exposed beyond their capacity. It becomes particularly evident when a clear object is moving in a dark field. All CCDs may be provided with on-chip mechanisms (anti-blooming gates) to drain away excess charges among columns in order to limit the effects of blooming. In cytometry, blooming must never be allowed to occur, and a good rule is to systematically avoid any excessive illumination of the sensor.

Photoelectrons in potential wells originating from incident photons are indistinguishable from thermal electrons freed from the silicon by thermal agitation. Thus, each photoelement read out consists of signal (electrons originating from photons) and noise (non signal or 'dark' electrons).

Noise originating from the silicon photoelement is called *dark current* and increases with thermal agitation, that is to say chip temperature. At room temperature, thermal noise may generate thousands of electrons per pixel per second and is a concern for long-lasting low light exposures. By and large, each 10°C of cooling halves the dark current. Cooling the device to −60°C or below reduces dark currents to levels as low as 1 electron per pixel per second (Aikens *et al.*, 1989).

The architecture of CCD sensors mounted on video cameras is dictated by the need for the image-sensitive area to be masked and thus shut off from light when the charges are moved row by row to the serial register to provide the output (Aikens *et al.*, 1989). The simplest architecture is the full-frame CCD sensor where an electronic shutter blocks incident light when charges are moved to the serial register. However, this architecture is not common in image cytometry cameras of any type.

The CCD architecture commonly found in scientific video cameras is the frame-transfer CCD (*Figure 2.3*). Here, a second parallel register

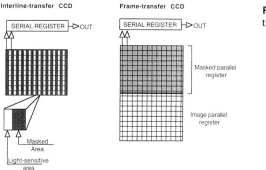

Figure 2.3. Architecture of frame-transfer and interline-transfer CCD.

that is permanently masked from the light is arranged in tandem with the parallel register used for the image array. Therefore, we have two identical CCD sensors, one of which serves as a storage area that temporarily collects charges during read out, thereby eliminating the need for an optical shutter. The shift across the CCD chip from the image array to the storage array takes from 400 µs to 1 ms, depending on the size of the CCD sensor. When charges in the storage array are read, the image array can again collect light. Although not a common practice, the storage array can also be unmasked and both CCD sensors can be used to collect large images, provided that a shutter mechanism is then in use, as is the case in full-frame CCDs.

A frame-transfer CCD is an effective but costly solution, because CCD wafers are expensive. Therefore, the interline transfer CCD (*Figure 2.3*) was developed for industrial and domestic but also for scientific video cameras. This configuration combines two parallel registers into a single array at the expense of light efficiency. Indeed, part of each photoelement of an interline transfer CCD is masked by electronic circuits that form an image storage register during read-out: the image area of interline transfer CCDs consists of vertical light-insensitive or storage columns alternating with light-sensitive columns of photoelements. The vertical columns form the interline mask that behaves like the storage register in the more expensive frame-transfer CCDs. Therefore, the area available for light collection is reduced to less than 50% of the actual CCD chip. For this reason, interline transfer CCDs have a rather low sensitivity to photons and are not practical for low light conditions, such as fluorescence or luminescence. On the other hand, transfer of charges from an exposed pixel column to the adjacent masked column is very fast, requiring only a couple of microseconds.

The photoelement portion exposed to light in a CCD sensor is expressed as a percentage of its total area. A *fill factor* of 100% indicates that the entire photoelement surface is exposed to light. A fill factor of 32% indicates that only 32% of the surface of a photoelement is available to sense light. The remaining portion is covered by the interline mask or other electronic elements, such as anti-blooming gates.

Loss of spatial resolution due to the presence of the interline mask in the image array is not that important and interline transfer CCDs of scientific or industrial grade are commonly used in video cameras for image cytometry when transmitted light or bright fluorescent images are captured.

CCDs vary greatly with respect to physical dimensions and number of photoelements. CCD sensors mounted in video cameras are usually rectangular or square chips with sides ranging from 3.5 mm to over 35 mm. The individual photoelements are rectangular or square units whose sides range from 6 μm to over 20 μm.

> *Photoelement dimensions* are calculated by dividing the length of the chip side by the number of photoelements in a row or column. In an 8.8 × 6.6 mm chip with 756 (H) × 582 (V) photoelements, a photoelement measures 11.6 × 11.3 μm. In interline transfer CCDs, the dimension of the photoelement sensing area is obtained by multiplying these numbers by the fill factor (e.g. by 0.32). 'H' indicates the number of photoelements in a row and, hence, the number of CCD columns, and 'V' indicates the number of photoelements in a column and, hence, the number of CCD rows.

For planar calculus, it is convenient to have square photoelements in the CCD, but this is not a strict requirement for image cytometry. Larger sensors acquire larger images whereas smaller photoelements allow larger spatial resolution. Conversely, large photoelements are more sensitive to light and collect larger amounts of electrons. The saturation charge in electrons (also known as 'full well capacity') is approximately 1000 times the photoelement light-sensing area expressed in square microns (Aikens *et al.*, 1989). For this reason, low-light applications preferentially require sensors with large photoelements and 100% fill factor that are maintained at low temperature to avoid dark current and to increase the dynamic range of the device.

> The *dynamic range* is a property of image sensors that depends primarily on photoelement dimensions, but also on silicon substrate and temperature of the chip. The dynamic range of a single photoelement is the ratio between the number of electrons collected in the potential well at saturation and the number of electrons liberated from the silicon by dark current. Therefore, the dynamic range is increased either by enlarging the size of the photoelements so that they can collect more electrons, or by cooling the sensor to decrease dark current. However, the dynamic range of an imaging system in practice must also account for all the noise sources other than sensor dark current. Dynamic range can be expressed as a ratio of either the number of electrons at full well capacity and the number of electrons produced by dark current, or else signal intensity at saturation and signal intensity in the dark. Alternatively dynamic range can be given as the equivalent decibel (dB) rating. For example, a saturation to dark current ratio of 100 000 electrons:50 electrons results in a dynamic range of 2000:1 equivalent to $20 \times \log_{10} 2000 = 66.02$ dB.

Manufacturers grade sensor quality from 0 (top quality) to 3 (low grade) by determining lack of uniformity per individual pixel or per grouped pixels in the image plane. Usually, pixel nonuniformity is defined under uniform illumination at 50% saturation (for an 8 bit signal, this is at the 128 gray level) as the difference in luminance between a single photoelement and the average value of the photoelements within a selected neighborhood. Pixels deviating 5% or more from the average value are defined as bad pixels or blemishes. Manufacturers of scientific sensors classify CCD chips according to a blemish map, which is obtained by recording the number of defects in the form of points, clusters or entire columns or rows. Top quality sensors cost more, obviously. Since objects that are measured in image cytometry are usually covered by many pixels, the tolerance in cytometry is quite high, and bad pixels do not form a problem, because they are only one of many and do not disturb measurements.

As we have mentioned previously, the efficiency of CCD sensors to generate electrons from incident photons, or quantum efficiency, is in general very high throughout the visible part of the spectrum (*Figure 2.4*).

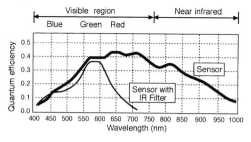

Figure 2.4. Quantum response of a CCD sensor (Kodak Kaf-1400) over the visible spectrum.

Quantum efficiency of 1:1 or 100% means that an electron is formed for every photon reaching the photoelement. In the visible region of the spectrum, CCDs have a high quantum efficiency, but less than unity.

The incoming light hits the photoelements from the front, where all the electronic connections and polysilicon gates are positioned. These polysilicon connections are hardly transparent at wavelengths shorter than 400 nm. Therefore, special thinned CCDs have been constructed with a ~15 μm thin silicon substrate to increase quantum efficiency at short wavelengths (*Figure 2.5*). Thinned CCD sensors are illuminated from the back and are not commonly used in image cytometry.

CCD sensors are very sensitive to infrared radiation and when working in visible light an infrared blocking filter should always be interposed between the light source and the chip to avoid blurred images and high levels of noise (Jonker *et al.*, 1997).

Charge injecting device sensors. Charge injecting device sensors are silicon detectors that are similar to CCDs in their general structure, and which can also be used as imagers in video cameras. The main difference resides in the nondestructive read-out of the photoelement charges. When charges are read out from a CCD chip, either the incoming light is

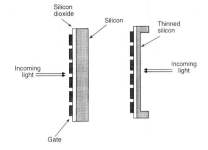

Figure 2.5. Front and retro-illuminated CCD. Reproduced from Aikens *et al* (1989) Solid-state imagers for microscopy *Methods in Cell Biology* **16**: 291–313, with permission of Academic Press.

blocked or charges are transferred to a light-masked storage register. In both cases, photoelements are fully depleted of electrons and the image is erased. In CID sensors, charges are shifted between electrical connections *within* the photoelement, and it is the amount of displacement that is determined and forms the output. Therefore, charges can be read at various intervals without blocking light and depleting the potential wells. In this way, it is possible to monitor and elaborate images during exposure. This operation can be done at the single-pixel level, because photoelements of CID sensors are individually addressed. Images are erased by 'injecting' charges in the silicon substrate in which the photoelement is buried, instead of 'transferring' charges to the row above. Another property of CID sensors is their inherently superior anti-blooming performance. Indeed, light overloads remain confined to the individual photoelements without spilling over to the nearby elements. These features of CIDs increase the dynamic range of the sensor and allow accurate acquisition of both weak and intense optical signals in the same exposure cycle. Although image cytometry makes much more use of CCDs, CIDs provide a useful alternative, in particular for fluorescence studies where bright and faint objects coexist in the same image.

Complementary metal-oxide semiconductor devices. In the introduction to a technical article describing CCD sensors, Morley M. Blouke and co-workers at Texas Instruments Inc. and Jet Propulsion Laboratory wrote in 1983 'The principal motivation for the rapid development of large area CCD imagers has, of course, been the desire to fabricate a fully TV-compatible, all-solid-state imager on a single chip'. Less than 20 years later, the entire camera and not only the imager can reside on a single chip that directly interfaces with a TV monitor. This is made possible by CMOS. CMOS devices collect light over an image area that is, similarly to CCDs and CIDs, made up of thousands or millions of radiation-sensitive photoelements distributed in rows and columns. However, CMOS photoelements do not accumulate the electrons generated as charge packets in a potential well, but behave as photo-diodes where the reverse current varies with illumination, continuously creating a voltage that is read at the end of the integration period.

Semiconductor photodiode arrays were developed in the late 1960s even before CCDs were invented, but in the early days they had a series of limitations such as the absence of a gain function in the photoelement, significant noise problems and severe nonuniformity caused by the parallel nature of the photodiode array. It was the limited performance of these early semiconductor diode arrays that led to huge investments in CCDs. The real breakthrough with CMOS sensors came with the re-examination of these problems and the development of on-chip active compensation techniques. In particular, the active pixel sensor (APS) technology, which was developed in the early 1990s, utilizes an amplifier (gain) for each photoelement. Other on-chip technologies, such as correlated double sampling or active column sensor, substantially reduce noise. Although CCDs were first developed for the most demanding applications, such as astronomy and microscopy, before moving into the industrial and home markets, CMOS-APS devices were developed due to commercial need for low-end digital cameras for mass consumption on the one hand and for highly miniaturized low-power radiation-resistant imaging systems by space agencies on the other.

The structure and the properties of the CMOS image plane, however, are not very different from those of CCDs and CIDs. In scientific imaging, the use of CMOS is destined to increase for the following reasons:

(i) Unlike CCDs and CIDs, which require custom fabrication equipment and are thus expensive, CMOS sensors can be manufactured economically on standard semiconductor fabrication lines.

(ii) Since CMOS sensors are made in semiconductor factories, their design can be easily standardized on a world basis and the additional circuitry necessary for image handling, such as analog to digital conversion, digital signal processing, shuttering and automatic exposure control, windowing, color interpolation and image compression, can be built into the same chip that is housing the image plane.

(iii) Unlike CCDs, which shift electrons through nearby photoelements to the output amplifier, each photoelement in a CMOS has its own amplifier and output. Tasks such as sub-array imaging by random access (also known as 'windowing') are much easier to implement and increase the read-out speed dramatically.

(iv) CMOS sensors are low-power devices.

(v) Because polysilicon is not needed anywhere in the photoelement, the quantum efficiency of CMOS in the blue region is much higher than that of CCDs, and photodiodes can profit of the full range of silicon light transparency from 200 to 1100 nm.

(vi) The dynamic range in CMOS devices can be very high, up to 1 000 000:1 (120 dB or 20 bits in a single exposure) because a processor compresses the signal output logarithmically at each pixel, reducing both blooming and over- or underexposure. A logarithmic output may not at first glance seem to be a desirable property for image cytometry. However, as we will show in Section

4.3.4, the signal can be made linear by calibrating output with the use of a few neutral density filters of different ODs.

Color CMOS camera-on-a-chip devices are being developed at the moment with built-in audio at prices lower than U.S.$200, including a front lens. At present, the overall quality and performance of CCD and CID sensors are still better than those of CMOS sensors, particularly when a high fill factor is necessary. Commercially available CMOS devices are still small and mainly developed to provide miniaturized consumer video cameras at low cost. However, the image quality of CMOS sensors is quickly catching up with that of CCDs, so that in most cases one can see hardly any difference between images produced by these systems with the naked eye.

Today, most microscope image analysis systems use framegrabbers coupled to either a CCD imager or, when a high dynamic range is required, to a CID imager. However, image cytometrists should be aware of developments in CMOS technology. In the future, it will probably be possible for laboratories to have a different CMOS device for each task (photometry, fluorescence, large areas, high-definition imaging, etc.). The CMOS devices can all be connected to one computer through a single port, and it will be easy to switch from one to another.

2.1.2 Imagers

For use in an image cytometry system, a silicon chip imager has to be assembled into a package that allows the sensor to be effectively placed behind a microscope objective. The assembly comes in the form of a camera that is commercially available. Irrespective of the sensor type mounted, the choice of the camera requires a set of decisions: (i) video or still camera; (ii) analog or digital output; (iii) industrial or scientific camera; and (iv) monochrome or color.

Video and still cameras. As the names imply, video cameras are designed to capture moving scenes, whereas still cameras shoot 'still' pictures. Video and still cameras belong to two separate commercial sectors in the consumer and industrial arenas, but in image cytometry this distinction is much less marked. Both cameras use a solid-state sensor as photoplane and both are capable of delivering high-quality images. Video cameras, which came on the market much earlier, are the most widely used imagers by cytometrists and allow imaging of living objects in real time.

Still cameras for top-level photomicroscopy mostly work via a computer connection. Manufacturers of still cameras generally emphasize the final appearance of the image by providing fine color balance and compensation features as well as great morphological details, and this is what you pay for. The highest quality still cameras for microscopy incorporate a cooling mechanism to deliver brilliantly clear images of low-light-level specimens, such as multicolor fluorescent images. Still microscopy cameras use a single CCD and proprietary opto-mechanical mechanisms to provide non-interpolated color images of high quality. This mechanism functions by quickly alternating red, green and blue (RGB) filters in front of the sensor and shooting three images in rapid succession. The three images are digitally converted by the camera electronics and the software reconstructs a full color image (see below) that is sent to the computer. Therefore, it takes at least a second to generate a complete image and the observer cannot obtain a real-time image at the highest resolution on the monitor. However, it is possible to see in real-time a low-resolution color or monochromatic image, either on the computer monitor or on a small liquid crystal display mounted on the camera.

Very high definition images are not required in routine cytometric work. In assembling a system for image cytometry, for planar, photometric or stereological analysis, the choice to be made is monochrome or color. When photometric measurements are necessary, a monochromatic video camera with fine light adjustment and calibrated light response is mandatory. Color still cameras can be used by cytometrists for planar measurements and stereological work, but video cameras perform these tasks equally well.

Analog and digital output. Still cameras are able to memorize images on a memory card or diskette that can be successively read by a computer. This way of imaging is not commonly employed in image cytometry where cameras are mostly connected to a computer via a cable so that images can be seen on the computer monitor in real time. Therefore, cameras used in image cytometry have an output cable through which image data flow to the computer. The signal coming from the amplifier of the solid-state sensor is always a linear sequence of electrical impulses. In analog output cameras, the electrical signal travels through a coaxial cable to the computer where it is digitized. In digital output cameras, the signal is immediately digitized in the camera, so that only binary impulses have to travel along the connecting cable to the computer.

A *coaxial cable* is a copper wire transmission line centered inside an insulator surrounded by an outer metallic mesh which serves both as a second conductor and as an electromagnetic shield. It is used for transmission of analog video signals.

In analog output cameras, the signal may be a standard or nonstandard video signal, where spatial information is converted to time delays in the electrical signal and light intensity is converted into the amplitude of the electrical signal (i.e. volts). The image analysis system of camera, cable, framegrabber and computer constitute a closed-circuit TV (often referred to as CCTV), that shares some of the properties of wireless broadcast TV.

Standard video signaling follows official committee recommendations (e.g. the Electronics Industry Association or EIA in the USA) that set engineering standards specifying timing frequencies, timing-pulse voltages, field rate in Hz etc. In black-and-white cameras, the video signal carries only light intensity information (luminance) and the mostly widely used standards are RS-170 (in the USA) or CCIR (in Europe) for broadcasting TV and RS-330 for closed-circuit TV. In color cameras, video signals also carry color information (chrominance) and the most widely used standards are NTSC in the USA and PAL in Europe. All signals are defined as 'composite', because the electric impulses carrying luminance information are combined with sync pulses of reverse polarity which separate the signal into segments (*Figure 2.6*). Each segment between two sync pulses of the signal corresponds to approximately a horizontal line (pixel row) of the active image area.

In the RS-170/NTSC standards, each video frame is subdivided in 525 time portions (horizontal lines) of which 483 are used for image representation of the scene and the remaining 42 portions are used for synchronization (timing) purposes. Video frames are repeated 30 times per second. Likewise, in CCIR/PAL standards subdivision is in 625 time portions, of which 576 are used for image representation and 49 for timing purposes. Video frames are repeated 25 times per second. However, when images are presented to the human eye at frequency lower than 40 Hz (i.e. 40 cycles per second), an annoying sensation of flicker is perceived. Thus, field interlacing was adopted in TV systems to enhance frequency without increasing the bandwidth of the transmission system. The scene is scanned in two fields, the odd and the even.

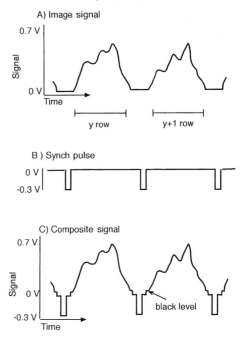

Figure 2.6. Composite video signal. The analog signal between two sync signals contains brightness information of a photoelement row. Reproduced from Inoué (1986) *Video Microscopy*, with permission of Kluwer Academic/Plenum Publisher.

The odd field consists of every other horizontal line (1st, 3rd, 5th etc.), and the even field consists of the even lines (2nd, 4th, 6th etc.). The alternating fields are then recombined in the final image, the frame. This scanning method is called '2:1 interlace' and is an economic way of reducing flicker, since fields can be scanned 60 or 50 times per second depending on the standard (*Table 2.1*).

Table 2.1. Summary of specifications of broadcasting standards

		RS170/NTSC	CCIR/PAL	Formula
A	Lines/frame	525	625	
B	Frames/s	30	25	
C	Lines/field	262.5	312.5	A/2
D	H scan rate	15 750 Hz	15 625 Hz	$C \times B$
E	H scan interval	63.5 μs	64 μs	$1/D \cdot 10^6$
F	Vertical frequency (fields/s)	60 Hz	50 Hz	$B \cdot 2$
G	V-scan interval	16.67 ms	20 ms	$C/D \cdot 10^3$
H	Active scan lines	483 lines/frame	576 lines/frame	$A -$ blank scans
G	Aspect ratio	4:3	4:3	Width:height

As far as image quality is concerned, all these standard signals are equivalent. Therefore, only a few aspects need to have the attention of the image cytometrist:

(i) The RS-170/NTSC and the CCIR/PAL standards determine that images are captured into an active image area resolved by 483 or 576 horizontal lines, respectively. In both cases, pixel rows in the sensor exceeding this available space in the video signal are left out. Images captured with the American standard are smaller in terms of the number of lines than those taken with the European standard.

(ii) The signal of the video camera must be digitized by a framegrabber card that accepts the standards of the output of the video camera.

(iii) According to the video standards mentioned above, a pixel is considered to be square when the width of the active image area in the sensor and on the monitor is 1.33 times its height, or in other words when the image aspect ratio is 4:3. Images must conform to this standard for reproduction to occur without geometric distortion, such as circles appearing as ellipses. When displayed on a VGA computer monitor, common 4:3 formats for an image in pixels are 512×384, 640×480, 768×576, 800×600 and 1024×768.

Interlaced scans that do not conform to these specifications and progressive scans are nonstandard video signals, which are used in applications where very high resolution, large image dimensions, fast motion and/or on-chip integration are of prime importance.

Progressive scan is now an emerging standard of video format which reads out (or displays on a monitor) all the image data in a sequential order, one line at a time from top to bottom, in such a way that one field equals one frame. For instance, computer monitors as well as professional analog monitors and new TV monitors are progressively scanned. Computer monitors are addressed by an internal video card that behaves as an interface which adjusts all video signals entering the computer to the correct format. Professional scanned monitors can also display interlaced signals as the monitor electronics will transform them into progressive signals.

A progressive scan imager is mandatory for applications that cannot tolerate the time difference between fields of interlaced video. This is rarely the case in image cytometry where images are not captured of moving objects, although it may be obligatory for applications measuring photon emission in the range of microseconds, as in time-resolved microscopy (Marriot *et al.*, 1991). Because the acquiring of a progressive scan image by a framegrabber is simpler than the use of interlaced signals, and progressive scan monitors present much less flicker than interlaced monitors, progressive scan technology has rapidly evolved. As living cell cytochemistry is developing fast, the recording of moving objects will become an important application of this approach.

A few things must also be kept in mind by the image cytometrist when considering nonstandard video signals:

(i) All architecture types (full frame, frame transfer or interline transfer) support either interlaced or progressive scan video signals, although solid-state chips are designed for a specific scanning mode. A progressive scan image sensor may also deliver interlaced signals, but its design is not optimized for this.

(ii) Progressive scan is linked to the bandwidth of the system. A video camera or a monitor can use progressive scan to a given resolution and use interlaced scanning when higher resolutions are required.

(iii) A frame transfer rate to the monitor higher than 20 Hz (20 half-interlaced fields or 20 full progressive frames per second) is required to obtain images in a satisfactory live-mode.

Whatever the standard or format, an analog video signal is a sequence of electrical pulses that must be transformed into computer-readable numbers before being transmitted to and memorized in the computer RAM. Therefore, the output of a video camera is transmitted through a coaxial cable to a special computer board, known as a framegrabber or digitizer, which has special electronic circuits that sample the analog signal at given intervals and translate it into a digital form.

We have already discussed how a video signal is formed by lines of analog information, which last a certain period of time and are separated from the previous and following signals by sync pulses. The full amplitude range of a video signal is 1 V, where 0.7 V is used for the luminance information in the image and 0.3 V for sync pulses. The white saturation signal is reached at +0.7 V. A framegrabber with a standard video signal input is designed to know perfectly when the active image area starts in the standard video signal and how to separate the single lines. Thus, framegrabbers are provided with a pixel clock that allows the signal of every line to be dissected.

The fundamental mechanism implemented in framegrabber boards is the analog to digital (A/D) converter that reads the luminance value at each interval and transforms it into a luminance number, which is referred to as gray level (*Figure 2.7*). In this input/output function, the resulting value is proportional to the luminance at that interval. The lowest output value (0) indicates no light and the highest output value (255 for an 8 bit depth digitization) indicates signal saturation (0.7 V). For an RGB color image, this operation is performed three times in parallel, whereas for a composite color video signal, a second A/D converter reads chrominance values. It is here that the term 'pixel' starts to appear particularly appropriate. The framegrabber transforms each point of the image into an image element that takes a digital gray value so that the image can be transmitted as numbers to the computer memory.

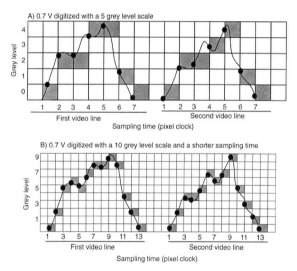

Figure 2.7. During the analog-to-digital transformation in the framegrabber, the A/D converter assigns a numerical value proportional to the voltage of the signal (brightness) at a frequency determined by the pixel clock.

In image cytometry, A/D converters are second in importance only to imager photoelements. Their pixel clock can either be fixed at a given frequency or else be software-programable, and the higher the frequency (in MHz), the larger the number of pixels retrieved in a video line. The phase locked loop (PLL) is a timing mechanism commonly found in framegrabbers. It locks in into the sync signal and subdivides the continuous analog video signal into partitions each of which represents one discrete pixel in the computer memory. In high-resolution imaging, PLL accuracy, which is measured in nanoseconds, determines the fidelity in matching the photoelements of the imager.

Matching pixels: the video sync signal establishes the number of lines (or the height) of an image and the framegrabber establishes how many pixels form one line (*Figure 2.1*). The optimal situation is reached when the number of framegrabber pixels matches the number of photoelements in the imager rows. When the framegrabber sampling frequency allows less pixels than sensor photoelements, the image will be undersampled with consequent loss of image information. In the reverse situation, the image will be oversampled and of no use because in that case the photoelement is the least resolvable unit in the image.

Another important factor is the number of values that the A/D converter can assign to gray levels or bit depth. Today, most image cytometry studies are performed with a bit depth of 8 (256 gray levels or 2^8 bits). However, greater depth is preferable when it is necessary to examine details in dark or bright objects in one image, such as in low-light applications, or when a high degree of photometric accuracy is required to measure dark objects. However, greater depths also require higher board processing speed, improved power dissipation and a more critical management of nonuniformity and noise by the A/D converter. Today these aspects are well under control and most framegrabbers offer a 10 bit or 12 bit depth, corresponding to 1024 (2^{10} bits) and 4096 (2^{12} bits) gray levels. The bit depth should approximate the dynamic range allowed by the signal-to-noise ratio (S/N) of the camera (see p. 26). A sensor with a 50 dB S/N allows a $10^{50/20}$=316:1 dynamic range and may be satisfactory coupled to a 2^8 bit A/D converter. A 72 dB S/N sensor allows a $10^{72/20}$=3981:1 dynamic range and should be coupled to a 2^{12} bit A/D converter.

In assigning gray levels, A/D converters have to maintain the same timing and interval length along the full range of luminance to reproduce exactly the photo response of the imager. For instance, an ideal 4 bit A/D converter should divide the 700 mV range of luminance transmitted by a linear response imager into 16 gray levels, where any digit combination (0000, 0001,... 0111 ... 1111) represents a 700/16 = 43.75 mV range of luminance. To do this, the least significant bit (LSB) changes (i.e. from 0 to 1 or vice versa) occur at fixed time intervals, say 80 ns, thereby incrementing the code. Differential linearity errors arise when a certain degree of variability in the association code-luminance appears along the signal intensity curve, causing nonlinearities in the output. This is called *differential nonlinearity* (DNL). Details in the image will then no longer be resolved at the full bit range, i.e. 4 bits in this example. The LSB may fluctuate as an error without contributing to the reproduction of the original information. The term *pixel jitter* indicates those alterations that are caused by DNL when the information carried by one or more of the LSB in the pixel code is degraded and thus fails to reproduce the original details of the object. When this happens, the waveform distortion becomes particularly evident due to irregularities present when imaging thin straight lines. In an A/D converter, DNL or pixel jitter should not exceed $\pm\frac{1}{2}$ LSB or ±10 ns.

Another relevant mechanism to be considered in a framegrabber is the frame transfer rate, that is the speed at which the image is transferred to the computer RAM memory. This speed depends on the set of chips of the framegrabber, the computer bus transfer rate, the main processor speed, and the type of RAM chips. When the rate at which data are captured is faster than the rate at which the system can handle them, a certain amount of on-board buffer memory is needed to handle the overflow resulting from the speed mismatch.

Frame transfer rate is given in megabytes per second (MB s^{-1}) and is calculated as image width × image height × number of color channels × bytes per color × frames per second. The theoretical speed of the peripheral component interconnect (PCI) parallel bus to which most of today's framegrabbers interface is 132 MB s^{-1}, but the effective bus bandwidth ranges from 40 to 80 MB s^{-1}. With the advent of PCI fast computer buffers, many framegrabbers have access to the computer main board either in a direct memory access (DMA) mode or in a unified memory architecture (UMA) mode. DMA transfers data to normal computer RAM memory, whereas UMA transfers data to a video-dedicated RAM memory space, when present in the host computer. Both transfer modes bypass the main processor. In addition, framegrabbers may transfer data to the memory of the video display card, which is linearly mapped in the computer main processor. Whatever the selected mechanism, image data are displayed after they have been digitized and made available for processing.

Besides capturing images and transferring them to the computer memory, framegrabbers are able to perform many image processing functions, including image compression, in real time, directly on the board hardware. However, for image cytometry, computer-based processing is preferable, whereby the computer main processor performs the processing tasks on digitized images. In this case, the framegrabber serves only as a camera interface and acquisition device for transferring images to the computer as quickly and accurately as possible.

A *basic principle* in image cytometry dictates that data coming from the measuring device (imager) should flow unmodified into the computer RAM memory. Therefore, on-board digital signal processing (DSP) and image compression should be avoided in image photometric work and may be used only for simple planar measurements after accurate spatial calibration.

Besides basic compatibility with the computer hardware and with the imager, only a few details must be kept in mind when selecting a framegrabber for cytometric studies:

(i) The process of capturing images from nonstandard sources requires a board with a high-frequency programable pixel clock.

(ii) The supported frame transfer rate for noncompressed images should provide at least 20 fields per second (20 fps) to permit live video display from the video source.

(iii) For routine cytometric work using standard video signals, low-cost 8 bit monochrome framegrabbers with a fixed pixel clock may prove satisfactory, provided that they do not introduce uncontrolled image processes, such as data compression, automatic gain control or nonlinear gamma (see below).

(iv) The framegrabber should be associated with demonstration programs and with a macro language, a software library or a developer kit containing all the functions and source codes needed to control the hardware, which can be easily implemented into custom software.

(v) Whatever the selected framegrabber board, it has to pass benchmark tests (see Chapter 4) and has to be calibrated before it can be used for image cytometry.

Digital output cameras are made up of two devices housed in a single case: the imager and the framegrabber. A/D conversion is performed inside the camera module and the data are digitized pixel by pixel as they flow off the sensor amplifier. Only digital information (as opposed to the analog video signal) travels along a cable to a proper interface card in the computer. The presence of A/D conversion close to the sensor, however, produces heat and therefore additional energy dissipation mechanisms are needed to keep dark current low.

One advantage of using an analog output is that a single framegrabber can be connected to several different imagers, so that a number of imagers may occupy a single computer slot. In contrast, depending on the type of interface, digital output cameras today require an interface and slot for each imager. In the very near future, however, multiple digital cameras may be connected to the same high-speed IEEE 1394 or USB 2.0 serial busses. Currently, IEEE 1394 ('DV', 'Firewire' or 'iLink') interfaced cameras can deliver up to 400 Mbits s^{-1}, allowing real-time display of images on the monitor. The development of USB 2.0 promises to deliver the same read-out speed, while the next generation of IEEE 1394 is designed for 1600 Mbits s^{-1}.

A benefit of digital output is that the accuracy of data can be optimized for the particular sensor type that is used by the camera and, once digital, the information cannot be degraded by cabling. Usually, digital cameras have better quality circuits, lower noise, higher sensitivity and superior dynamic range then standard analog cameras. Only high-end scientific grade analog cameras are of comparable quality.

Major features of a digital output camera are the following:

(i) The A/D conversion clock is synchronized with the sensor clock, thereby eliminating pixel jitter.

(ii) It is always possible to read the amount of brightness of an image in gray levels in real time.

(iii) Various camera functions such as gain and gamma control subarray scanning, on-chip integration and pixel binning (see below) are standard on most digital output cameras.

(iv) All the above functions can be controlled via software by the user in real time. Benchmark tests and calibration are easily and quickly performed.

Industrial and scientific video cameras. The largest dilemma today when setting up an image cytometry system regards the choice of video camera. Is a good quality industrial video camera sufficient for image cytometry or is a scientific camera necessary? And if we opt for a scientific camera, do we need a high-definition or a cooled camera? A decision of this sort can easily make a difference of several thousand dollars. It is therefore essential to gain practical understanding of the basic elements that are necessary to perform our studies validly and on which a proper choice depends.

We do not need to consider the consumer or home cameras that are usually produced as camcorders or small low-priced cameras for displaying images on a TV monitor or VCR. The entry point for cytometric tasks is an industrial, surveillance or machine-vision type camera.

> It is not a simple matter for a cytometrist to acquire a video camera module or a sensor from the original manufacturer! Indeed, most sensors and cameras are available only for the *component* or original equipment manufacturers (OEM) market where companies sell large amounts of units. This means that they may not be readily available for the end consumer.

In general, cameras contain an image module that can be attached to the microscope via a C-mount type of connection and go with a separate power supply that feeds the module via a cable with low-voltage DC current. The dividing line between scientific and industrial cameras is not clear-cut. Many camera modules use the same CCD sensor and the distinction between scientific and industrial cameras may depend on the electronics built in the module around the sensor. A typical example is the monochrome Sony XC77/ce camera module, which has been on the market since 1991: it was initially used for a wide variety of industrial, machine-vision and microscopy tasks but it was also introduced in high-performance microscopic analysis systems (C72 series Dage-MTI, Michigan City, IN, USA).

Industrial cameras can have either an analog or a digital output. They are built around a standard format solid-state sensor, usually of the interline transfer type. The standard solid-state sensors that are mounted on industrial cameras are rectangular, representing the familiar 4:3 aspect ratio of standard television. The sensor format is defined as $\frac{2}{3}$, $\frac{1}{2}$ or $\frac{1}{3}$ inch, but it should be noted that these values do not refer to the actual physical size of the sensor. They merely indicate that the camera may be used with optics and lenses matching the corresponding diameter of the frontplate of thermionic cameras. It is a convention to provide compatibility with lenses and optical distances of old thermionic tubes. The lens size has to correspond with the imager format: a camera with a $\frac{2}{3}$ inch sensor, which measures 8.8×6.6 mm, should be used with a $\frac{2}{3}$ inch lens.

Smaller formats and sizes offer better value for money and camera designers are able to reduce the size of CCD sensors for reasons of cost and miniaturization without greatly sacrificing performance. For example, the $\frac{1}{3}$ inch sensor of a CCIR camera is 4.8×3.6 mm and has a resolution of 752 (H) $\times$ 582 (V) photoelements, thus each photoelement turns out to be as small as 6.5×6.25 μm. The interline architecture of these sensors reduces the fill factor still further. Although small pixels may provide a large spatial resolution, when they have a fill factor lower than 0.5, their ability to sample light is considerably compromised. This problem can be solved by 'on chip lens' technology, first developed at Sony in 1992 with the name of Hyper-HAD™ (hole accumulated diode), incorporating a tiny condenser lens over each pixel which increases photoelement sensitivity to light.

In the future, camera formats larger than $\frac{1}{3}$ inch may not be produced anymore in the consumer market and will be offered only as component/OEM devices.

A $\frac{2}{3}$ *inch sensor* mounted on the microscope through a C-mount covers a satisfactory large area at the middle of the objective field of view. Smaller sensor sizes cover smaller areas and may be inadequate for image cytometry. Intermediate (relay) lenses can be interposed in front of the sensor, usually mounted inside a C-mount, to reduce the objective primary image and allow the sensor to cover a wider part of the field. However, relay and on-chip lenses may increase light scattering and glare phenomena and may interfere with the accuracy of photometric work.

Scientific-grade high-end imagers are still largely analog output devices (although digital output scientific cameras have now started to appear) using large CID or CCD sensors of the highest quality with full-frame or frame-transfer architecture. The video signal is of the nonstandard progressive type. The main difference between these scientific-grade cameras and their industrial-grade counterparts lies in the higher dynamic range and lower thermal noise of the former type. Although the basic properties of high-quality imagers, such as photo response and quantum efficiency at different wavelengths, are the same as those of industrial grade imagers, scientific video cameras are provided with electronic circuits that optimize the control of sensor functions and noise. Two main types of scientific grade video cameras are manufactured: (i) high-definition large sensor cameras; and (ii) low-light cameras.

The first type is built around sensors with an array of 1024×1024 or more square photoelements of small dimension ($\leqslant 8.0$ μm) to obtain large images with high definition.

The second type, the low-light camera, is built around smaller sensors with photoelements of larger dimensions (> 20 μm) and is cooled to sub-zero temperatures with a Peltier-mechanism or helium. These cameras are used for low-light conditions where it is necessary to accumulate photoelectrons for many seconds or even minutes, such as in fluorescence and luminometry microscopy and astronomy. Low-noise cameras exist that are designed to acquire low-light digital images at speeds of 500–1500 images per second and these are used in real-time physiology to trace the flow or the spectral modifications of fluorescent probes in living cells and tissue and in time-resolved microscopy. High speeds are reached by speeding up the A/D conversion, by limiting the image to a small subarray in the sensor or by increasing the sensitivity of the sensor through binning.

> The technique known as *'binning'* combines a block of pixels into a single super pixel. Thus, sensitivity and dynamic range are increased because the light-sensing area of a number of photoelements is associated and the read-out is faster because the reduction in the number of rows diminishes the amount of information transmitted.

To increase dynamic range, scientific-grade video cameras have to be coupled with a high-quality framegrabber in order to achieve an optimized management of system noise. It has already been demonstrated that dark current is kept low by cooling the camera. However, the heat of the on-chip output amplifier also adds noise (pre-amplifier noise) to the signal. The best way to reduce that is to slow down the read-out, as is done by low-light integrating cameras. Both dark current and pre-amplifier noise lower the dynamic range of the system by increasing the black level (signal value at zero incident light), thereby interfering with the accuracy of photometric measurements at low light. The total noise (NT) may be calculated in electrons as

$$NT = \sqrt{NP^2 + NE}$$

where NP are the electrons produced by pre-amplifier noise and NE electrons produced by dark current (Aikens *et al.*, 1989).

On top of these sources of noise, other sources also exist that add or mix up electrons in the signal, as already has been discussed in relation to DNL in the A/D converter. These types of noise include the effects of the quantum nature of light (photon noise), the process of frame transfer on the CCD chip (transfer noise), and the pixel nonuniformity in the chip (scene noise). These forms of noise do not systematically add electrons to the signal, but affect the LSB of the code by increasing variability (for an extensive discussion of the different forms of noise in image cytometry, see Aikens, 1990; Chieco *et al.*, 1994; Jonker *et al.*, 1997).

> The *signal-to-noise ratio* (S/N or SNR) of a video system is established by the manufacturer and summarizes the range of the system response to changes of light. It includes most of the above-mentioned forms of noise and may be expressed either as a S/N ratio or in dB in a similar way as for the usable dynamic range.
>
> *Scene noise*, which is related to systematic photoelement-to-photoelement variation in dimension, offset and gain, can be determined by the user in small uniform subregions of the image at various levels of illumination as the mean pixel gray level divided by the standard deviation in gray level values (Tsay *et al.*, 1990; Chieco *et al.*, 1994).

Camera systems usually are provided with a series of mechanisms to control incident light and signal output. These may or may not be useful for image cytometry or may even hinder validity in cytometry (Chieco *et al.*, 1994; Jonker *et al.*, 1997). Some of these mechanisms have already been discussed.

It is useful to summarize the items that we are likely to come across in camera specification sheets:

(i) *Sensor architecture* – economical interline transfer sensors are commonly used for image cytometry, although the frame-transfer devices that are usually mounted in scientific cameras allow higher dynamic ranges.

(ii) *Sensing area* – with industrial-type cameras a $\frac{2}{3}$ inch sensor is optimal for image cytometry. With scientific cameras, the choice is application-dependent.

(iii) *Picture elements* – the higher the number of horizontal (H) elements (columns), the better the image definition. The higher the number of vertical (V) elements (rows), the larger the image dimension. In general, industrial-type cameras have an H resolution higher than 750 (H) elements, and this should be matched by a proper framegrabber clock frequency in order to avoid loss of image definition.

(iv) *Pixel size* – pixels may be rectangular or square. The square pixel format is better suited for applications where rotation transformations have to be applied to images. Photoelement sides should be smaller than 12 μm for high-resolution image cytometry and larger than 20 μm for low-light image cytometry.

(v) *Fill factor* – in full-frame and frame-transfer devices the fill factor approximates 100%; in interline transfer CCD sensors the fill factor drops to 25–40%. The higher the fill factor, the higher the dynamic range of the sensor.

(vi) *Saturation signal* – the saturation signal indicates the number of electrons in a potential well at saturation.

(vii) *Signal system* – interlaced (EIA or CCIR) standard video signals are commonly used in image cytometry with industrial-grade cameras. Progressive scans are mainly used for monitoring moving objects and are standard in scientific-grade cameras. Since progressive scan signals are simpler and provide better results, they will also become standard in industrial cameras in the not too distant future. Several interlaced cameras also provide noninterlaced scans by transmitting only the odd or even fields with an evident loss in V resolution.

(viii) *Binning number* – a binning number shows whether it is possible to use the binning mode to produce superpixels. It indicates the size (in pixels) of a superpixel ($2 \times 2, \ldots 8 \times 8$ etc).

(ix) *Pixel addressing* – pixels may be addressed individually as in CID cameras, allowing superior dynamic range, speed and sensitivity.

(x) *H/V resolution* – in conventional terms, camera performance is often expressed in H or V TV lines, as a result of a test performed with an EIA resolution chart. These specifications indicate the maximum number of horizontal or vertical lines that can be discerned in an image (resolving power). The higher these numbers are, the better the image definition. The values depend on the number of sensor lines and rows and on noise management by the electronic circuits of the camera.

(xi) *Output connectors* – for monochrome industrial cameras, video signals are usually transferred through a coaxial cable with a BNC connector to the framegrabber or an analog monitor. Color cameras may have an additional D-sub RGB connector through which the separate RGB signals are transferred. Digital cameras use appropriate digital cables to transfer the digitized signal to a computer interface or to an RS-232 compatible serial port.

(xii) *Exposure/integration time* – for analog-output industrial cameras, exposure integration time is determined by the standard signal. In digital-output and in scientific-grade cameras it may range from less than 1 ms to more than 1 min. Exposures longer than 5 s require proper cooling of the sensor.

(xiii) *Signal to noise ratio (S/N ratio)* – S/N ratios are usually expressed in decibels. S/N ratios or cameras for image cytometry should be better than 50 dB or 300:1.

(xiv) *External synchronization system/external trigger/gen-lock/ asynchronous scanning* – these mechanisms are mainly used to synchronize the signal with that of other cameras or with an external event or reference. Triggering can be used in image cytometry, for example, to prevent bleaching in fluorescence studies by recording images with time lapse exposure.

(xv) *Lens mount* – for industrial cameras, the lens mount should be of the C-type to facilitate the connection to the microscope. Scientific cameras with a different mount require proper connecting tubes to the microscope.

(xvi) *Clock out* – clock out is expressed in MHz and indicates the frequency of the pixel clock that is used for reading a row. The higher the number of photoelements, the higher the frequency must be. Its value enables synchronization of the A/D converter with the timing of pixel read out.

(xvii) *Time delay and integration (TDI)* – TDI synchronizes the row by row transfer of charges in the sensor with the movement of a moving object and is mainly used in machine-vision applications. Not used in routine image cytometry.

(xviii) *Electronic shutters* – electronic shutters are on-chip electronic devices that regulate the intensity of light by quickly obscuring the photoplane. For a standard signal camera, shutter speed is normally set between 1/25 and 1/60 s, but it can be switched to a faster speed down to 1/10 000 s or more. Electronic shutters are adopted mainly to image fast-moving objects or to decrease light intensity under bright conditions. They are not commonly needed in image cytometry where images do not move and light is under strict control. However, they may be useful in time-resolved fluorescence if synchronized with a rotating chopper plate in the microscope, although there are situations where the use of an additional computer-controlled mechanical shutter may be preferable.

(xix) *Gain* – the light responsive amplitude of the composite video signal ranges from 0.3 V, the level corresponding to a zero light signal or dark current, to 1.0 V, the level corresponding by default to the pixel full well capacity. It is this 0.7 V spanning luminous signal that is digitized in gray levels by the A/D converter. The 1.0 V level is under the control of the gain set of the video camera or framegrabber. To meet the need for high light sensitivity, it is possible to increase the gain of either the camera by assigning a 1.0 V output level to a nonsaturated pixel capacity, or of the framegrabber by instructing the A/D converter to assign the maximum gray level available to a voltage less than 1.0 V. In either case, A/D conversion reaches saturation faster and thus increases the gray level resolution at low light, and hence sensitivity. Conversely, to meet requirements of a high signal-to-noise ratio when small differences in intensity have to be measured over a bright background, gain has to be reduced. In the video camera, the default setting, commonly reported as $1 \times$ or 0 dB, spans the full 0.7 V range that is optimal to reach the highest dynamic range. In commercially available cameras, a higher gain can be selected with a switch in +6 dB steps, each corresponding to a $2 \times$ gain or a one-f stop lens aperture.

It is important to be aware that, with increasing gain, noise is increased and dynamic range decreased.

(xx) *Automatic gain control (AGC)* – AGC is a feature that is used in most commercially available video cameras to automatically scale the electrical output to the brightest area of the image. It may be useful for color imaging when using different objectives. In image cytometry, AGC must always be switched off for photometric purposes.

(xxi) *Offset* – offset, also referred as bias, pedestal or dark level indicates the voltage assigned to the dark current when the sensor is not illuminated. In the composite video signal it is usually set at 0.3 V. In scientific video cameras, it can be increased to avoid spurious signals or background noise (such as autofluorescence). In cytometry, it is more common to modify the offset via software either by instructing the A/D converter to start digital conversion at a higher level of the signal, or by subtracting a dark level image from all digitized images.

(xxii) *Gamma correction* – the signal output of a monochrome CCD camera should respond linearly to the illumination of the faceplate when AGC is switched off and the exponent of the function that relates the output signal to the input signal, or 'γ', is set to 1. When transmission has to be read directly from pixel brightness, a $\gamma = 1$ ensures an output voltage that is linear with the input signal. When the γ control of the camera is switched on, γ decreases to approximately 0.45 and hence the output is no longer linear. This γ compensation was originally introduced to match nonlinearities in monitor response (Inoué, 1986; Aikens *et al.*, 1989). As outlined in the section on calibration (see Section 4.3), a $\gamma<1$ can be a desirable feature for quantitative cytochemistry with nonscientific-grade cameras because it provides additional gray levels at high absorbance values, thus extending the dynamic range of the device.

Monochromatic and color cameras. Video cameras are monochrome or color. For photometric studies, it is necessary to use a monochrome camera, but planar and stereological measurements can be performed with color images.

To produce a video signal with color information, video and still cameras mostly use the RGB color system. The RGB system is based on the principle that an image is collected with incident light filtered through a red filter, a second image through a green filter and a third image through a blue filter. Thus, three color component images or 'channels', each of which is monochromatic, are retrieved. After image processing they provide a single full-color image. The RGB system produces color images in a similar way to that by which cone photoreceptors in the retina produce color images on the basis of red, blue and green as the three primary colors of human vision (Castleman, 1998).

Three major principles are used in video cameras to reproduce RGB color images:

(i) In the most economic setup, each photoelement in the sensor is covered by a tiny red, blue or green filter in a 'mosaic' or 'vertical' stripe manner. Color is then reconstructed by the camera electronics by interpolating the light information from groups of three or four differently RGB filtered photoelements in a single pixel at the expense of spatial resolution. When a color pixel is derived from photoelements filtered using a four-element scheme (Bayer pattern), two green filters are used on one diagonal, because the human eye is most sensitive for green. Although the effective spatial resolution of the sensor is reduced, color images of high quality can still be retrieved because several sophisticated 'tricks' are implemented in or around the sensor to reduce loss of spatial resolution. Loss becomes evident only when images are enlarged (color aliasing).

(ii) In another setup, the camera uses three identical image sensor chips, namely one for each primary color. Behind the lens of the camera an RGB color-splitting prism is placed that sends three identical images to the three different sensors. Interpolation is not necessary with this design as images maintain the full spatial resolution of the sensor, thereby allowing optimal image quality and enabling top quality color images in live mode. However, the use of three sensors and the complex design make these video cameras rather expensive. In microscopy, 3-chip color cameras are used in video systems where the video signal is directly sent to an analog monitor for teaching and discussion. It is rarely used in image cytometry.

(iii) A third design, which is generally implemented in still cameras and scientific video cameras, uses a wheel with the three color filters in front of a single sensor. The camera captures three pictures in rapid succession and reconstructs a full-resolution RGB color image. This design produces very high definition color images under bright or low light condition (as for example occurs in multiple labeling fluorescence) with either standard or scientific CCD sensors. Because real-time imaging requires >20 images per second, a full-resolution image can usually not be obtained in live mode, particularly when large sensors are used. Indeed, the wheel movement requires time and the amount of information transferred from scientific sensors may be too large to allow live-mode speed through the cable. Therefore, with this design, live mode can be obtained only in a monochromatic or a low-resolution color mode.

To obtain a good color balance on the monitor, all video cameras have automatic and/or manual white compensation mechanisms that allow the user to set the white. It is commonly a simple button on the side of the camera, called 'white balance' that has to be pressed over an empty area. This is done once when the camera is switched on and after the light setting in the microscope has been optimized.

Cameras used in image cytometry, whether monochromatic or color, produce at least 8 bit depth images, that is images with $2^8 = 256$ gray levels. Each of the three color component images in the RGB color system therefore has an 8 bit depth. Their combination produces images with $256^3 = 16.8$ million different colors.

2.2 Microscope

In image cytometry, the imager is mounted on a microscope. Images may be obtained from any sort of light microscopy (transmission, fluorescence, dark field, polarization, phase or interference contrast, or confocal). The microscope may be upright, inverted, compound or stereo. Whatever microscope is used, the faceplate sensor is usually positioned by a proper coupler at a point where the primary image plane formed by the objective is located. No eyepiece lenses are interposed between the objective and the sensor, although a compensating eyepiece in the tube is necessary when lateral chromatic aberration is evident in color images or in images taken at two wavelengths, with a large distance in between (Bartels and Thompson, 1994; Inoué, 1986).

Most video cameras have a standard female C-mount attachment for lenses that also allows the camera to be connected to the microscope. The vertical dimension of the male C-mount coupler in the microscope is calibrated to permit the sensor to be positioned exactly in the primary image plane. The C-mount adapter, which is usually empty, may harbor relay lenses that reduce the image. A reduced image may be necessary when the video camera has a small sensor that covers only a small part of the field of view of the objective. In addition, a reducing relay lens may be used in combination with a low-power (1–2.5 ×) objective to allow imaging of large objects (e.g. an entire tissue section). It is useful to keep a spare (0.5–0.65 ×) reducing C-mount at hand which can be used when needed.

Cytometrists usually do not have a lack of experience with a microscope and are able to optimize illumination (as explained in several teaching manuals: Inoué, 1986; James and Tanke, 1991; Lacey, 1989; Pluta, 1988). Only a few details need emphasis.

2.2.1 *Illumination pathway*

Proper illumination is the key to success in image cytometry. Microscope illumination setting and adjustment must assure a uniformly illuminated field of view under any condition. Proper Koehler alignment, which is necessary because filament lamps produce light with uneven intensity, avoids vignetting and saves a great deal of work, because nonuniformly illuminated images have to be software-corrected before most of the procedures of image analysis can be employed.

With transmitted light microscopy, it is advisable to use at least a 12 V 100 W tungsten halogen lamp, which requires an external lamp housing, due to the high working temperatures generated (>250°C). A powerful light source is necessary because colored filters or relay optics interposed in the light path decrease the light intensity. The lamp should be connected to an external stabilized DC power supply with a very fine light intensity regulation and a clearly visible digital LED display where the current or voltage can be easily read. A DC power supply stabilizes light flux, eliminating noise and flicker from AC power lines.

For incidence fluorescence illumination, high pressure 50–100 W mercury (Hg) or xenon lamps are commonly used that are connected to their own power supplies, which do not allow light adjustment.

2.2.2 *Viewing tube*

The trinocular viewing tube of the microscope should include three beamsplitter positions. One position transfers all light to the binocular viewer, interrupting the light flux to the camera. A second position divides the light flux 50–50 between camera and viewer, allowing the image to be observed simultaneously with the eye pieces and on the monitor. The third position transfers all light to the camera, which is necessary when working at low light levels with the sensor in integrating mode.

A photographic reticulum should be mounted inside one of the two eyepieces of the binocular. The reticulum will help to match the focus plane of the image with that of the sensor.

2.2.3 *Objectives*

A set of objectives, including low-power lenses (1–2.5 ×) for measuring dimensions of large objects or entire sections, and mid-power lenses (6.5–40 ×) for operative measurements of microscopic objects, cover most of the needs encountered in image cytometry. For cytometric studies using transmitted light, it is not necessary to use expensive objectives; it is sufficient that the objectives are planar in the area captured by the sensor such that the entire field of view is in focus. At low-power (up to 10 ×) resolution of microscope objectives is far better than that of top-level video cameras. At mid and high power, the resolution of the camera matches that of the objectives, and lens quality may affect image sharpness and contrast.

The tiny pixel sizes of solid-state imagers guarantees a measuring spot small enough to allow the use of mid-power objectives for both photometric and morphometric work. Costly high-power highly corrected immersion objectives (65–100 ×) are necessary only for a few types of analysis, for example when studying chromosomes or intracellular organelles (e.g. lysosomes or mitochondria).

For photometric measurements, it is essential to have the entire thickness of the object in focus. The depth of field can be calculated as

$$\text{Depth of field} = \frac{n\lambda}{\text{NA}^2}$$

where n is the refractive index of the object space (air, $n=1$ or oil, $n \sim 1.5$), λ the wavelength of the light in microns, and NA the numerical aperture of the objective. Objectives with 20–40 × power and small numerical aperture (NA) are usually satisfactory (Chieco *et al.,* 1994; James and Tanke, 1991; Pluta, 1988).

When an objective is selected, major points to consider are chromatic and spherical aberrations and glare. The most expensive objectives are of the apochromatic type that correct for differences in diffraction of light at various wavelengths. This correction avoids small changes in image focusing when objects are viewed either with white light or with monochromatic light at different wavelengths. It should be stressed here that, no matter how costly they may be, objectives should always be tested in practice at the bench. We have found that low-cost achromatic objectives can perform satisfactorily, whereas costly apochromatic objectives may require corrective optics in the tube.

Glare or stray light is an aberration of microscope objectives that may be extremely relevant for image cytometry (Chieco *et al.*, 1994). The term 'glare' indicates diffuse light that originates from the empty background of the scene and falls on the objects present in the image, increasing their apparent transmission. This aberration is a serious concern for photometric work, but does not significantly affect planar or morphometric measurements, except for a decrease in contrast in the image. Glare originates from reflection and scattering of light on glass–air surfaces, and therefore increases with the number of lenses introduced in the objective. This means that glare should theoretically be higher in the more complex and corrected (and thus more expensive) objectives. However, due to modern lens coatings, the equation 'high complexity = high glare' does not always hold true. Unfortunately, the degree of glare affecting objectives is not reported by the manufacturers and therefore this aberration can only be evaluated at the bench (see Section 4.3).

2.2.4 Motorized microscope stages

Although not absolutely necessary for performing cytometric measurements, a motorized microscope stage is highly advisable. In the early days of cytometry, motorized stages were used to quickly scan single cells and nuclei with a tiny light spot in a raster manner, a function that

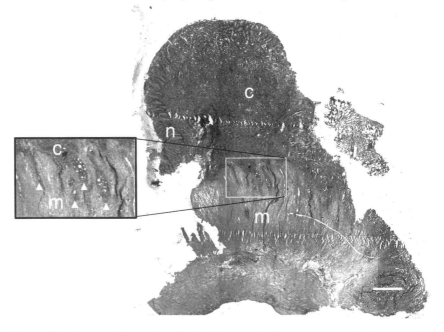

Figure 2.8. Composite large-size digitized image of an entire section of a human colon cancer that was made by sampling a series of images using a mid-power objective and a motorized stage. In this way, a large-sized image with high spatial resolution is obtained (see insert, zoom in of a detailed area in the section). The image was kindly provided by Dr Angela Köhler, Hamburg, Germany.

is now no longer necessary because objects are electronically multi-sampled by the sensor photoelements. However, motorized stages may be connected to a computer through a standard RS-232 interface and software controlled for x, y and even z coordinates. Motorized stages are directed with a few simple commands that can be easily implemented in user software to randomize sampling in histological and cytological preparations. A motorized stage can be useful for sampling series of images of a tissue section to stitch images to obtain composite larger sized images (*Figure 2.8*; Schmitt and Eggers, 1999). Random sampling is also carried out easily with a motorized stage. It is of fundamental importance for statistically correct and reproducible analysis and can also save time and effort (see Section 3.2.2). Unfortunately, motorized stages are expensive pieces of equipment. This is a reason for the cytometrist to make a careful and realistic assessment of what equipment is really required. When a lot of money is wasted on an unnecessarily sophisticated camera, framegrabber or microscope objective, there may be no money to spend on a motorized stage.

References

Aikens, R.S. (1990) CCD cameras for video microscopy. In: *Optical Microscopy for Biology* (eds B. Herman and K. Jacobson), Wiley-Liss, New York, pp. 207–218.

Aikens, R.S., Agard, D.A. and Sedat, J.W. (1989) Solid-state imagers for microscopy. *Meth. Cell Biol.* **16:** 291–313.

Bartels, P. and Thompson, D. (1994) The video photometer. In: *Image Analysis. A Primer for Pathologists* (eds A.M. Marchevsky and P.H. Bartels), Raven Press, New York, pp. 29–56.

Boyle, W.S. and Smith, G.E. (1970) Charge-coupled semiconductor devices. *Bell Syst. Technol. J.* **49:** 587–593.

Castleman, K.R. (1998) Concepts in imaging and microscopy: color image processing for microscopy. *Bol. Bull.* **194:** 100–110.

Chieco, P., Jonker, A., Melchiorri, C., Vanni, G. and Van Noorden, C.J.F. (1994) A user's guide for avoiding errors in absorbance image cytometry: a review with original experimental observations. *Histochem. J.* **26:** 1–19.

Inoué, S. (1986) *Video Microscopy*. Plenum Press, New York.

James, J. and Tanke, H.J. (1991) *Biomedical Light Microscopy*. Kluwer Academic, Dordrecht.

Jonker, A., Geerts, W.J.C., Chieco, P., Moorman, A.F.M., Lamers, W.H. and Van Noorden, C.J.F. (1997) Basic strategies for valid cytometry using image analysis. *Histochem. J.* **29:** 347–364.

Kristian, J. and Blouke, M. (1982) Charge-coupled devices in astronomy. *Sci. Am.* **247:** 48–55.

Lacey, A.J. (ed.) (1989) *Light Microscopy in Biology. A Practical Approach*. IRL Press, Oxford.

Marriott, G., Clegg, R.M., Arnd-Jovin, D.J. and Jovin, T.M. (1991) Time resolved microscopy. Phosphorescence and delayed fluorescence imaging. *Biophys. J.* **6:** 1374–1387.

Pluta, M. (1988) *Advanced Light Microscopy*, Vol 1. *Principles and Basic Properties*. Elsevier, Amsterdam.

Schmitt, O. and Eggers, R. (1999) Flat-bed scanning as a tool for quantitative neuroimaging. *J. Microsc.* **196:** 337–346.

Theuwissen, A.J.P. (1995) *Solid-State Imaging with Charge-Coupled Devices.* Kluwer Academic, Dordrecht.

Tsay, T.T., Inman, R., Wray, B., Herman, B. and Jacobson, K. (1990) Characterization of low-level cameras for digitized video microscopy. *J. Microsc.* **160:** 141–159.

3 Software

Image cytometry software does not need to be complex. It must guarantee good, straightforward interactivity to help the user to isolate the objects of interest and to conduct reliable measurements.

Three major types of software are needed in image cytometry: software for image acquisition (see Section 3.1); software for image analysis (see Section 3.2); and software for data collection and number-crunching (see Section 3.3). Accessory software for the control of filter wheels, choppers and motorized stages is often integrated in image-acquisition software.

3.1 Acquisition software

Video-capture software is associated with a specific acquisition hardware and is based on proprietary programs (device drivers) which are necessary to guarantee compatibility with the operating system (e.g. DOS, Windows, Mac OS, UNIX, etc.). Various framegrabbers are associated with ready-to-use software modules, called plug-ins, that allow acquisition and display of images from other well-known image analysis or image processing programs. Most manufacturers of framegrabbers and digital output cameras have a software development kit (SDK) available for programers. These SDKs contain a set of routines, protocols and tools that enable a programer to build specific software applications. These development kits have been of great importance in image cytometry since the late 1980s because they allow customization and control of image acquisition. Initially, programs for image cytometry were constructed in the laboratory with the use of SDKs and were usually unique for a single type of frame-grabber or platform. Their basic architecture, which was generally developed for the DOS platform, was designed to provide a fast way to acquire and analyze images because the small storage capacity of computer mass memory disks at that time meant that it was not practical to save images.

Nowadays both hard disks and removable disk drives have huge storage capacities which continue to increase. The concepts for image analysis software have therefore changed in line with the development of new video systems and computer platforms. The wide variety of cameras, framegrabbers and other camera-computer interfaces (i.e. IEEE 1394 Fire Wire and USB2 serial busses) now available and in continuous development has made it desirable to have acquisition and camera control functions (easily implemented with the SDKs given by the manufacturer) independent of image analysis software. This strategy avoids restrictions and delays due to incompatibilities between software and hardware. It is now possible to use SDKs to build up acquisition software for each device that is available. Indeed, today there is a continuous flow of more and more simple tools for constructing software applications, such as new multimedia standard formats (e.g. Microsoft's 16 bit Video for Windows and 32 bit Direct Show, and Apple's QuickTime™) and application format interfaces (API). In the Windows operating environment, the Direct Show protocol (part of a set of software libraries grouped under the name of DirectX) includes an extensive number of application format interfaces, making it easier for a programer to develop capture applications that have access to the hardware features of framegrabbers.

Both the in-house-developed and the manufacturer-provided acquisition software require inclusion of only a few easily implemented routines that make it possible to display and calibrate images, as well as to acquire and save them rapidly.

In particular, image acquisition software should allow for:

(i) read-out in live mode of the intensity of image brightness (lowest, mean or modal and highest gray level or histogram display);

(ii) read-out of the mean or modal brightness of single small frames that are moved over the image to check for uniformity of illumination;

(iii) averaging of multiple frames;

(iv) easy switch to different acquisition modes (monochrome, color, etc.) and image sizes;

(v) drawing of reference points in displayed images;

(vi) saving images in different image formats;

(vii) rapid saving of sequential images with only a click of the mouse;

(viii) introduction of control commands for automatic movements, when a motorized stage on the microscope is available;

(ix) allowing for automated execution of steps of (i)–(viii), particularly useful for living cell cytochemistry.

The software that is available with digital output cameras usually allows γ, gain and other camera controls that have to be changed manually in analog output cameras to be changed.

3.2 Image analysis software

Image analysis programs are fundamental tools for the cytometrist (Adler, 2000). It is relatively straightforward, perhaps with the help of a knowledgeable professional, to build one's own image acquisition module, but this approach is not advisable for image analysis software, because it requires involvement of expert programers and analysts. Specific programs for cytometrists were developed in many laboratories in the early 1990s. Only a few of these programs became commercially available. The majority of the commercially available (and occasionally free-ware) image analysis programs that are available today is general-purpose software that includes built-in programing or macro-languages to automate sequential or repetitive tasks. These programs consist of various modules and tools to conduct single analysis (line or area measurements, gray level readings, binarization, etc.) that have to be organized in proper macro functions. The separation between image acquisition and image analysis software leaves the user free to select the most appropriate software for his/her needs.

In the following sections, we discuss one by one the essential features of image cytometry programs.

3.2.1 Calibration and measurement

Spatial calibration. Routines for spatial calibration should allow the cytometrist to construct and save a table to record the number of pixels in horizontal and vertical directions for a given length (usually in microns) and for a given optical setup (e.g. $10 \times$ objective, $25 \times$ objective or $25 \times$ objective in combination with a 0.65 relay lens). Once the table has been saved, the user should be able to switch rapidly from one setup to another. A different approach is used in some programs that calibrate only in horizontal dimensions and then require the pixel aspect ratio to be entered in order to calculate vertical dimensions. The end result is the same, but the first approach is more straightforward. Spatial calibration is used for calculations of lengths and areas.

Calculation of the *area* of an object is simple: identify the object and sum up the number of pixels that cover the object. The software converts, when required, the pixel number into absolute squared units (μm^2 or mm^2).

To measure the length of horizontal, vertical, or diagonal *lines* the user either manually traces the line with the help of the mouse or else uses software tools for autotracing the outline of an object. Straight lines may be manually traced but the tracing of *curves* and *perimeters* should always be software-assisted. The reason for this is clearly given by Barba *et al.* (1992): 'The number of points activated for the same distance is not the same for users because of different tracing speeds, and because most users will activate more points in an irregular curve than in a straight line. Likewise, a coarse tracing may activate neighboring points in a random zigzag manner. All these matters require consideration and treatment, before the tracing can be quantified'. In other words, a manually traced curve is a mess. For valid tracing, software has to be used. Correct length measurements can be obtained only when the soft-ware provides either autotracing tools that review and smooth a manually traced line or algorithms that extract one-pixel-wide contours of objects.

Although it might not be immediately apparent, the calculus to measure traced curved lines and perimeters is quite complex. As is shown in *Figure 3.1*, measurement of a straight line is just a matter of addition of pixels, but measurement of curved lines and perimeters requires detailed instructions with respect to the direction of each adjacent point of a curve (Joyce-Loebl, 1985). The user should be aware that routines for finding borders, edges or outlines of objects in image analysis programs show pixels around the objects, and their count is just a sum of areas in pixels and not the measurement of the actual length of the perimeter. In addition, we should also be aware that perimeter estimators are not stable, because perimeters of digitized objects vary with magnification: the measurement of a curved line segment increases as digitization becomes finer.

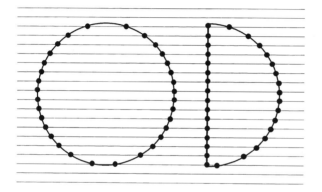

Figure 3.1. When a curved line or a perimeter is measured in a digitized image, it is necessary to account for the angle of each pixel with respect to the previous one on the line. A mere pixel count will not distinguish between a curved or a straight line.

A line segment may be considered as being digitized in *n* pixel points (each pixel has a definite size and thus may be considered to be a discrete vector). Therefore, a continuous line becomes digitized into a set of discrete vectors and thus its exact measurement is impossible. This means that lengths can only be estimated. Starting from the pixel at the beginning of a line, each neighboring pixel receives a code 'o' if it is orthogonal (90°) or 'd' if it is diagonal (45°) with respect to the previous one. Thus *n* codes lead to a *chain-code string*. The length of the digitized line equals the sum of pixel lengths. An 'o' pixel is given a smaller weight than a 'd' pixel, because pixels are larger in the diagonal dimension: if a line, say of 4 µm length, is covered by 100 horizontal pixels, it will be covered by 70 pixels only when it is turned diagonally. In either case, the measurement is affected by an error, and various authors have proposed different weighing schemes to reduce this error. The first proposed scheme is a weight of 1 for 'o' pixels and a weight of 1.414 (square root of 2) for 'd' pixels (Freeman, 1970). Note that many weight schemes were proposed for square pixels (1:1 aspect ratio), despite the fact that images are often composed of rectangular pixels. The software manual must clearly indicate the formulas adopted for line measurements.

Photometric calibration. When a video camera is used as a photometric head, its response to light has to be calibrated in transmission (T) or optical density (OD). As stated earlier, the signal output of CCD, CID and CMOS sensors responds proportionally with face plate illumination. Thus, if a limit is posed for maximal illumination, as is the case in a laboratory photometer, light intensities can be read as Ts and transformed into ODs using the Lambert–Beer formulas:

$$OD = \log_{10} \frac{1}{T} \text{ or } OD = 2 - \log_{10}\%T.$$

When the analog signal from a video camera is digitized, light intensities are transformed into gray levels that range from 0 to 255 when the framegrabber is provided with an 8 bit-depth digitizer or from 0 to 1023 when the digitizer is 10 bit. For quantitative photometric work, images have to be captured with monochromatic light. Thus, a monochromatic camera is sufficient. Three considerations should be borne in mind:

(i) It is important to check the bit depth with which the image cytometry software works. For example, the gray levels of a 10 bit image cannot be fully exploited with a software package that can handle only 8 bit images.

(ii) The software should provide one or more tables that enable the assignment of T or OD values to specific gray levels and the construction of a linear or polynomial regression line that will automatically transform gray levels into ODs. Since a different calibration table has to be created for each framegrabber and camera setup, and since it may be possible that gain or γ of the video camera has to be changed depending on the application, it is a good idea to save a number of calibration tables, one for every setup that we may introduce.

(iii) Last but not least, it is essential to make sure that the software transforms each individual pixel gray level of an object into OD before the output of the result of a photometric measurement. The procedure of single-pixel OD transformation has to be used to avoid distributional errors when measuring absorbance of irregularly stained objects, as is often the case in cytochemistry (Chieco *et al.*, 1994; Ornstein, 1952). The final photometric measurement may either be the mean OD or the sum of all ODs of every single pixel of the object (integral OD, or IOD). While mean OD is a measure of the concentration of an absorbing substance, the IOD is a measure of the total amount (mass) of absorbing substance in the object.

In fluorescence and luminometry studies, light is measured that is emitted by the object, not the light that is absorbed. Emission measurements do not suffer from distributional error and thus the mean gray level value of the light emitting object can be taken as final measurement, provided that emission intensities fall within the linear range of the video camera response.

Stereological tools. In cytology, planar morphometric measurements can be obtained easily with the use of stereological methods. Therefore, it is handy to superimpose commonly used stereological tools on the image, such as an unbiased counting frame (Gundersen, 1977) or a point-cross grid. These tools (*Figure 3.2*) can be overlaid either by means of computer graphics or by adding a second binary image of grids or frames.

Stereology was introduced in 1847 and was developed as an efficient discipline to obtain unbiased cytometric measurements of three-dimensional geometric features of objects from two-dimensional sections. Briefly, stereology is based on particular geometrical probes, frames, point grids and line grids of different complexities, which are super-imposed on an image. The count of the intersections of points and lines with the object of interest in serial two-dimensional sections allows measurements to be made of areas, boundaries and profiles, and translation of these measurements into volumes, surfaces and lengths, respectively. Before digital imaging, stereological probes were printed on transparencies that were overlaid on photographs or mounted as optical reticules inside the eye piece of a microscope. Nowadays, stereological frames and grids can be overlaid by computer graphics on digitized images and viewed on the monitor. The important point here is that stereological methods are based on solid mathematical and statistical foundations that allow generalization with respect to the entire specimen to be made from a few measurements performed in a number of small areas. Given the strong statistical basis of stereological measurements, a fundamental requirement is the ability to perform truly or systematic random sampling with respect to selection of fields inside a specimen and selection of objects within the field (for basic principles in stereology see: Gil and Barba, 1994; Howard and Reed, 1998).

3.2.2 Object and area selection

In image analysis, it is possible to either measure directly an object that is identified on the monitor or to mark the object and let the software do the measuring. When the software has to count the number of pixels and

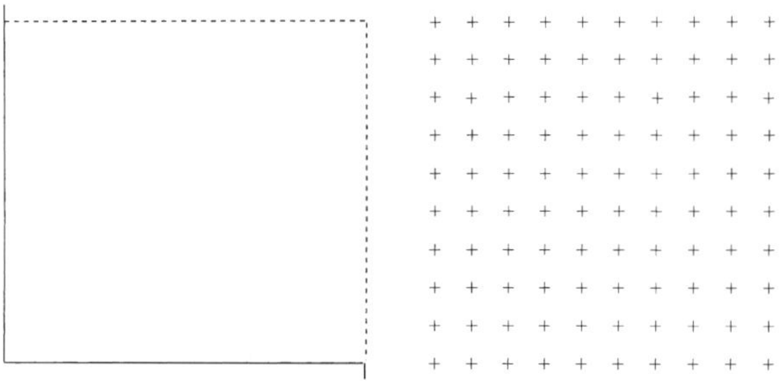

Figure 3.2. Unbiased counting frames (left) are used for object counting. Object profiles completely within the frame or intersected by dotted inclusion lines are counted. Any object profile touching the solid exclusion lines or the extension edges is discharged. Point grids (right) with cross-shaped points are commonly used to determine the area fraction of objects in an image. A point is considered a hit when the object profile covers the upper-right corner in the cross. To obtain the area fraction of the object(s) in the image, the number of points hitting object profiles is divided by the total number of points in the frame.

read out the pixels covering an object for the calculation of area, optical density, emission or shape factors, the user has to indicate the position of the object in the image. Image analysis programs provide tools for area selection and object selection to restrict the analysis to a particular area or object. All these tools may be moved or sized with the help of the mouse and are briefly described below.

Frames for area selection. Tools for area selection are used to overlay a rectangular, elliptical, polygonal or freehand frame, creating a subregion of the image. The subregion may consist of an entire object as such (e.g. a cell nucleus or a distinct area in a tissue section), or may simply limit further processing to an area where objects are located (such as a group of nuclei for DNA quantitation).

Binary segmentation and slicing for object selection. Traditionally, object selection is performed with the binarization procedure, which can be used only for objects that have a staining intensity that is sufficiently distinct from their surrounding. The user determines by trial and error an optimal gray level threshold that is higher than that of all or most of all object pixels and lower than that of the surrounding pixels or vice versa. Once the threshold has been set, the image is made binary; the identified objects are represented in black, and the background in white or vice versa.

A similar procedure is gray level slicing and involves creation of a range or a 'slice' of gray levels that include the feature of interest. With the slicing procedure, the user creates a lower and an upper gray level threshold limit to include the object. At the end of the slicing procedure, the objects maintain their original gray levels and the surrounding area is converted into background color. During measurement, only pixels with gray levels within the thresholds are considered.

Image analysis software should reserve the extremes of the gray level scale, 0 and 255 for 8 bit processing or 0 and 1023 for 10 bit processing for special purposes. The highest level of the scale, white, is reserved for setting the *background* gray level, which in most programs identifies areas that do not have to be analyzed or processed. The portion of the background in the image is thus effectively erased. The lowest level, black, is kept for setting the *foreground* gray level, to mark objects after binarization. Some types of software give the user the option of having white objects against a black background after binarization or to select different background or foreground colors.

Miscellaneous and automatic procedures. A useful tool for object and area selection is the 'eraser', which converts anything it touches to background. The feature of interest can easily be isolated by rubbing out all surrounding objects with the eraser.

Objects can also be identified by tools (e.g. a 'wand' tool) that automatically trace the edges of separate objects or subregions that share similar gray levels or color. The user clicks with the mouse on or near the object of interest and the program will then mark the edge of the object.

It is important to note that a truly *automated unbiased procedure* to select cytological objects in gray level or color images does not exist. Tools, like the wand, that appear to identify objects automatically, actually require instructions with respect to threshold criteria. The tools work well and save time when strongly contrasted objects are present in the image, but they cannot otherwise be standardized. As every cytologist or histologist knows, contrast of objects against the surrounding background may vary, even within a single preparation. A threshold that works fine with a well-contrasted object may work far less well when used in another area of the specimen. These difficulties arise when the object borders in a digitized image are not clear-cut. Borders and margins are always transition (high frequency) zones where confusion exists between whether the pixels belong to the object or the surrounding background.

A handy selection tool is the point counting procedure. With this procedure, the user moves a cursor over the image and counts objects by touching and marking them with a dot or some other symbol.

An object or feature is *segmented* when that object or feature has been identified by binarization, slicing or any other procedure whereby software automatically recognizes the object and discards its surrounding.

Once objects have been segmented, different software programs offer slightly different ways to proceed further, for example:

(i) segmented objects may be selected individually by a tracing tool (outlining). The software assumes that everything inside the outline belongs to the object.

(ii) Alternatively, segmented objects are automatically numbered by the program and measured separately.

(iii) A third system is based on a frame that is designed around each object to be measured in an image where the background has been segmented out by binarization, slicing or the eraser tool. The software assumes that all pixels in the frame that differ from the background belong to the object.

3.2.3 *Image processing*

Image analysis programs have a variety of routines for enhancing detail, improving colors, making illumination uniform and so on. However, the major goal of image cytometry is to measure objects and features, not to improve images, because this is really image processing. Indeed, modern microscopes generally guarantee well-contrasted and uniformly illuminated images that do not need extensive processing before they can be viewed and analyzed.

However, to speed up analysis, it is often necessary to identify objects clearly to allow the software to analyze them automatically. In that case, one must never forget that all final photometric, fluorometric or luminometric measurements have to be performed on gray values of pixels of the original digitized image. Therefore, when processing is required to identify objects, this must be done on a copy of the original image. Once identified, gray levels in the original image must be used for all photometric measurements. Thus, for cytometric studies, only a few processing routines are necessary.

Shading compensation. When a series of images is captured, it is useful to capture an empty field at the same time in order to compensate for illumination unevenness. Although modern microscope illumination alignments guarantee proper light distribution and video cameras capture only the most central area of the objective field (*Figure 3.3*), the periphery of the image may still be slightly darker than the center, especially when using low power objectives. This effect, which is known as 'shading', may introduce noise during object segmentation, particularly with poorly contrasted objects. An empty, so-called 'flat field', image collected under the same light conditions may be used to obtain a uniform light distribution in the image for optimizing object segmentation. Two algorithms are particularly useful for image compensation. The first uses a multiplicative formula performed in every pixel as:

$$\frac{(GL_{image})}{(GL_{flat\ field})} \times (modal\ GL_{flat\ field})$$

where GL is the gray level. The second formula subtracts GL in every pixel as:

$$(GL_{image}) - (GL_{flat\ field}) + (modal\ GL_{flat\ field}).$$

As for all operations that modify gray levels, compensation should not be performed on the original images used for photometric measurement.

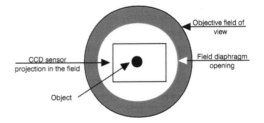

Figure 3.3. Correct position of the sensor projected over the objective field of vision. The rectangular image area must lie in the center of the field of view. The field diaphragm is then closed just around the measuring area to reduce glare.

Noise subtraction. Noise subtraction is mainly performed in the case of low-light images with relatively high background noise and low contrast, due to the use of long integration times during image capturing. Once an integration time has been established for the capturing process, a dark image without objects is captured and saved. The dark (or bias) image is then subtracted pixel by pixel from all captured images. Similarly, a weighted subtraction operation may be used to subtract autofluorescence from specific fluorescence as described by Van de Lest *et al.* (1995). Several framegrabbers and digital cameras provide background subtraction routines in the acquisition software.

Filtering. The term filtering refers to mathematical operations, technically defined as *spatial convolutions*, that change the gray level of every single pixel of the image on the basis of the gray level values of a given number of neighboring pixels. The group of pixels that is used to change the gray level of the central pixel forms a *kernel*; the weight given to each pixel of the group constitutes a *convolution coefficient*; and the array of coefficients constitutes a *convolution mask (Figure 3.4)*. Filtering is used on gray-scale, color or binary images. In gray-scale and color images, filtering procedures are mostly used to obtain smoothing (with low-pass filters) or sharpening (with high-pass filters) effects that attenuate background noise or enhance object details, respectively. Spatial filtering is not frequently used in image cytometry, and should be avoided when analyzing images that have been calibrated for photometric measurements.

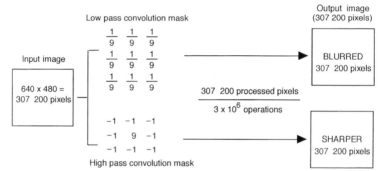

Figure 3.4. Commonly used kernel dimensions are 3×3 or 5×5 pixel arrays. Imagine that the convolution mask is placed with its central value over the pixel located at 892 (H), 560 (V) in the input image. The gray level of every pixel touched by the mask is multiplied by its respective coefficient and the multiplicands are summed. The result is placed in the output image at the same 892 (H), 560 (V) pixel location. This process is repeated for every pixel of the input image.

Contrast enhancement. Histogram stretching is the most common operation used for enhancing contrast and is obtained by multiplication or division of all pixel gray levels by a constant value. It is based on the gray level histogram of the image, a feature provided in all image analysis programs *(Figure 3.5)*. The captured image may sometimes include a limited number of the available gray levels. In such cases, the brightness ranges from light gray to dark gray and the image has poor contrast. The stretching process increases contrast of the image as it appears on the screen by rescaling the gray level values to the entire gray scale so that in the new image the lightest grays appear as white and the darkest as black. Equalization is an extreme contrast enhancement procedure used to uniformly disperse all gray level occurrences along the entire gray-scale histogram. Contrast enhancement is another operation that must never be used to modify memorized gray values of images that have been calibrated for photometric measurements.

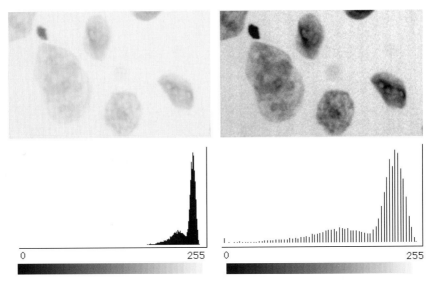

Figure 3.5. The gray level histogram is a graphical representation of the number of pixels for every gray level present in the image. The analysis of the histogram is informative for the evaluation of brightness and contrast of images, to determine how much of the available dynamic range is used by the image and to select a threshold value to distinguish objects from background. It may also be used to select an appropriate enhancement procedure. In the figure, a gray level image of Feulgen-stained cells (left) has been subjected to contrast enhancement using a histogram stretching function (right).

Binary image operations. Binary image operations are morphological operations and are used on binary images to improve the segmentation process by optimizing the image for automatic object recognition and measurement. Four binary operations are of value in image cytometry: opening, closing, outlining and skeletonization.

Opening operations remove small anomalies and background noise of binary images. Opening works sequentially, first by eroding pixels at the entire border of binarized objects and then by dilating the objects again with the same number of pixels. Tiny objects, such as points or spikes, that are background noise disappear during the erosion phase, leaving nothing to be dilated. At the end of an opening operation, the selected objects recover their original size and shape, but are cleaned up from noise.

A clean-up of binary images can also be obtained with routines that retain objects only when they are larger than a specified minimum dimension (e.g. 20 pixels). Another possibility is to employ an eraser tool for interactive removal of unwanted objects.

Closing operations remove small anomalies from objects in binary images. Closing works in the opposite way of opening. At all object/ background borders, objects are first dilated and then eroded. When a binarized object, like for instance a Feulgen-stained nucleus, contains small holes and gaps in it, the holes will be filled with black pixels, making the object appear completely black.

Similar results can be obtained when a painting tool is available in the software to interactively fill the holes with black.

Outlining operations are used to mark the boundaries of objects in the image.

Skeletonization erodes the black pixels in objects, leaving only a one-pixel-wide skeleton of every object. Symmetrical objects like squares or circles will be reduced to a single point, whereas asymmetrical objects like rectangles or ellipses will end up as a one-pixel-wide line marking the longest axis; irregular objects will produce branch-like lines. In cytometry, this operation is useful to convert elongated objects of variable size, such as bile canaliculi, vessels or alveolar lining, into one-pixel-wide lines so that length measurements can be made. A simple example is the visualization of the structural net of biliary canaliculi in liver lobules (*Figure 3.6*).

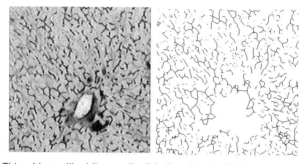

Figure 3.6. Thin objects, like bile canaliculi in liver lobule (left), may be shaped to single pixel width using a skeletonization procedure (right). A correct evaluation of the length of the canalicular net or of its staining intensity is possible only when the measurement is restricted to the canalicular skeleton.

Two-image operations. Mathematical (+, −, ×, :) or logical (AND, OR, XOR, NOT) operations can be performed on gray levels of corresponding pixels in two images or frames of the same size. The result is a third combined image. Because pixel values vary between two precise limits (e.g. 0 and 255 for 8 bit depth), we can decide to clamp results of the mathematical operations at the upper and lower limits of the gray scale. Alternatively, we may subtract 255 when the result is higher than 255; or add 255 when the result is lower than 0. A satisfactory understanding of the final effects of two-image operations may only be gained from practical experience. Other than for the already discussed shading compensation and noise or autofluorescence subtraction routines, in image cytometry operations on two images are only used in a few specific situations.

A two-image operation is used to convert the black pixels of an object in a binary image to its original gray levels while leaving the background white. This operation, which is known as *masking*, is a simple addition operation of gray levels to a black object with 0 gray value pixels.

Another two-image operation is used to add a stereological grid or frame to a target monochromatic or color image. The grid is drawn as a binary image containing a black grid over a white background or, else, a white grid over a black background. The black grid over white background is added to the target image using a logical 'AND' operation, The white grid over black background is added to the target image using a logical 'OR' operation.

> Image analysis programs are provided with an 'invert' function that inverts gray levels by subtracting them from the upper gray-scale limit. In binary images, black becomes white and white becomes black. In gray-level images, dark features become light and light features becomes dark. This command may help during two-image operations.

3.2.4 Image handling

With current image processing software, it is easy to modify image format, size and resolution. For analysis and calibration, attention should be paid to avoiding rescaling, compression or other changes that may distort measurements, and it is advisable to analyze images in their original size, format and resolution. All graphic formats compress data in some way to reduce file sizes when saving images to the disk. However, image compressed with lossless compression methods are bit-for-bit identical to the original when decompressed, while lossy compression methods always involve information loss. A basic color format used in image analysis is the 'bit-mapped' or 'raster' format, which in the Windows and OS/2 environments is abbreviated as BMP. Bit-mapped formats also include the PICT format for Macintosh, and the interchangeable lossless 'tagged image file format', abbreviated as TIFF, which in its native uncompressed format is not tied to any specific hardware.

Lossy compression algorithms and compressed image formats, such as the 'joint photographic expert group', or JPEG, are mainly used to reduce the total number of bytes for transmission or storage purposes. The compressed 'moving picture expert group' or MPEG is generally used to compress moving videos.

All the above formats handle binary, gray-scale and 32 bit color images, where 24 bits are used to generate 16 million colors and 8 bits are set aside for information details. Binary images require only one bit per pixel (with the value of 0 or 1), while gray-scale and color images require more than one bit and increase in size as the number of colors increases. Lossy image compression is not acceptable for storing raw images that have to be photometrically analyzed, but may be used for morphometric measurements provided that the format (e.g. 4:3) and the original size (e.g. 640×480) are maintained.

Besides image data, all formats provide a header detailing image width and height, color information, number of bits per pixel (i.e. 8 bit gray-scale or 3×8 bit = 24 bit color) and compression technique, if applicable. The storage sizes in bytes of common image formats are compared in *Table 3.1.*

Table 3.1. Size in kilobytes (kb) of a 640 (H) × 480 (V) image that is saved in different formats either in 24 bit color or 8 bit gray scale

Format	24 bit color (kb)	8 bit gray scale (kb)
BMP	922	308
TIFF	922	308
PICT	923	311
JPEG 100% quality	238	180
JPEG 50% quality	31	27

When images are opened by a program, color information included in the header is used to construct a 'look-up table' (LUT), which may be displayed beside the image or may be hidden to the user. A displayed LUT is simply a strip showing the shade of gray levels or the color assigned to each value of the gray scale. Commands, such as contrast or brightness modifiers, that modify the LUT of an image, change the image display and may also assign false colors to gray levels. Binarization is a command that changes the LUT by assigning black to pixels below the threshold, and white elsewhere. In most systems, it is possible to modify the LUT of the display only (hardware LUT), without modifying the values stored in the image memory. An 'apply LUT' command must follow a LUT modification of the image display to permanently modify the gray values of the stored image. In cytometry, it is good practice to save always a copy of the native image with its original LUT.

3.3 Data collection and number-crunching software

Data obtained from analysis may be recorded by hand or automatically stored in a table format inside a 'results window'. The entire content of the results table should be exportable to a text file and also remain available to be copied and pasted to other programs suitable for processing numbers and performing calculations. Image analysis software commonly employs a built-in programing language that can be used to add scripts and macros, to speed up routine procedures, to construct graphics, to automate complex multifunction tasks and to perform additional calculations (Russ, 1990). Dedicated software packages provide several calculations and graphics, such as those necessary for constructing DNA ploidy histograms or for pattern recognition. However, data arrangements in image cytometry are so variable that calculations and graphics are better performed by transferring measurements into spreadsheets or statistical software that is readily customized. Primary measurements in image cytometry are: counts, areas, lengths, perimeters, major or minor axis of objects, mean and modal gray levels, transmissions, mean ODs,

IODs, OD measurements along lines and profiles, and variances of pixel values. Additional shape and form factors can simply be derived from these basic measurements.

References

Adler, J. (2001) *Image Analysis*. BIOS Scientific Publishers, Oxford.

Barba, J., Chan, K.S. and Gil, J. (1992) Quantitative perimeter and area measurements of digital images. *Microsc. Res. Technol.* **21**: 300–314.

Chieco, P., Jonker, A., Melchiorri, C., Vanni, G. and Van Noorden, C.J.F. (1994) A user's guide for avoiding errors in absorbance image cytometry: a review with original experimental observations. *Histochem. J.* **26**: 1–19.

Freeman, H. (1970) Boundary encoding and processing. In: *Picture Processing and Psychopictories* (eds B.S. Lipkin and A. Rosenfeld). Academic Press, New York, pp. 241–266.

Gil, J. and Barba, J. (1994) Principles of Stereology. Computerized applications to anatomic pathology. In: *Image Analysis. A Primer for Pathologists* (eds A.M. Marchevsky and P.H. Bartels). Raven Press, New York, pp. 79–124.

Gundersen, H.J.G. (1977) Notes on the estimation of the numerical density of arbitrary profiles: the edge effect. *J. Microsc.* **111**: 219–223.

Howard, C.V. and Reed, M.G. (1998) *Unbiased Stereology*. BIOS Scientific Publishers, Oxford.

Joyce-Loebl (1985) *Image Analysis. Principles and Practice*. Short Run Press, Exeter.

Ornstein, L. (1952) The distributional error in microspectrophotometry. *Lab. Invest.* **1**: 250–262.

Russ, J.C. (1990) *Computer-Assisted Microscopy. The Measurement and Analysis of Images*. Plenum Press, New York.

Van de Lest, C.H.A., Versteeg, E.M.M., Veerkamp, J.H. and Van Kuppevelt T.H. (1995) Elimination of autofluorescence in immunofluorescence microscopy with digital image processing. *J. Histochem. Cytochem.* **43**: 727–730.

4 Calibration and benchmark testing

It is essential to calibrate and test the video microscopy system at the bench to make sure that the system produces valid measurement data. Solid-state cameras are stable sensors in comparison with older analog instrumentation, so it is generally sufficient to carefully examine the performances of a cytometric system and calibrate it at the bench when it is installed and when a given component is added or replaced. Only quick checks are necessary during daily working, mainly regarding light alignment.

4.1 Tools, targets and accessories

Calibration and benchmark operations are performed with the use of various sets of filters, targets and accessories. Some of these, such as bandpass filters, are used for operative measurements as well. With the term 'target' we mean calibrated geometrical figures and reticles in a glass slide or similar support that are used as precision standards for calibration, benchmark and quality control tests. All calibration and benchmark tools should be of absolute optical quality.

Stage micrometers. Stage micrometers consist of a reticle scale centered and mounted on a standard size glass microscope slide. The scale image is usually 2 mm long with divisions of 10 μm. It may have a one-axis (x) or two-axes (x, y) configuration. Stage micrometers are made by microscope or industrial optics industries under stringent manufacturing processes and quality control. In cytometry, stage micrometers are used for spatial or planar calibration to assign a length in microns to pixels and to assess the aspect ratio of images.

Graded neutral density filters. These are colloidal carbon gelatin or glass density filters calibrated to retain a set amount of light corresponding to a specified OD without altering the spectral characteristics of the light beam. The most popular OD gelatin filters, the Wratten series no. 96 manufactured by Eastman Kodak (Rochester, NY,

USA, www.kodak.com), can be cut to a desired size and mounted on plastic slide mounts for easy handling. The protective glass must be removed from the slide mounts carrying OD filters to prevent decreased transmittance. When inspected through a microscope objective, gelatin filters of highest densities appear somewhat grainy. Therefore, to obtain the most accurate calibration, the filters are positioned at the level of the field diaphragm below the condenser or above the objective, thus in a position where they can attenuate light without disturbing imaging. Filter size should be sufficiently large (2.5 cm diameter or more) to filter the entire light beam passing through the condenser.

Glass neutral density filters with anti-reflection coatings (Andover, Salem, NH, USA, www.andcorp.com; Balzers, Liechtenstein, www.btf.balzers.com; Edmund Industrial Optics, Barrington, NJ, USA, www.edmundoptics.com; Omega Optical, Brattleboro, VT, USA, www.omegafilters.com; Schott Glaswerke, Mainz, Germany) have similar properties to their gelatin cousins, but provide far better optical quality, because glass filters do not contain any visible particulates. The downside is that glass filters are much thicker and cannot be shaped or cut as can gelatin filters. On the other hand, glass filters can be positioned close to the light source, where gelatin filters melt.

Density-step gray-scale tablets with OD gradients along a strip are positioned at the specimen level and are convenient to determine a calibration range. Micrometer glass step tablets (Applied Image, Rochester, NY, USA, www.appliedimage.com) are preferred thanks to their high optical quality and ease of use.

In cytometry, neutral OD filters are used to:

(i) calibrate the photometric response of image sensors;
(ii) match the transmittance of different colored filters to ensure that the same light flux reaches the sensor under any given illumination;
(iii) reduce light flux to the sensor when using high power lamps whose light intensity cannot be adjusted.

Infrared blocking filters. Silicon sensors are oversensitive to infrared radiation. Therefore, a glass infrared blocking filter has to be mounted between light source and sensor (Jonker *et al.*, 1997a). It is best to have a glass infrared blocking filter at hand that can be positioned in the light beam of the microscope at least for three reasons:

(i) cameras do not always have an infrared blocking filter mounted;
(ii) it may be necessary to alternate measuring procedures requiring an infrared blocking filter with procedures that do not require it (e.g. when measurements require infrared light);
(iii) an infrared blocking filter should always be interposed as the first filter in front of a high-power light source, such as those used for fluorescent work, to reduce heat.

Infrared passing filter. Infrared passing filters are glass or gelatin filters that transmit light only with wavelengths higher than 700 nm. In cytometry, they are used to exclude counterstaining while imaging with a CCD sensor to count solid particles, such as silver grains in photographic emulsions.

Bandpass filters. Interference or band pass filters transmit only light of a given narrow band of wavelengths. They are made of glass. Depending on the manufacturer or filter type, the transmitted light has a half-peak bandwidth of 6–15 nm around a nominal wavelength. The larger the bandwidth, the higher the amount of light transmitted, and the lower the wavelength selectivity. They are positioned between light source and object, usually at the level of the field diaphragm. The filters should be large enough (2.5 cm diameter or more) or have a proper black chassis to prevent any spurious nonmonochromatic light entering the condenser.

Cytometry requires the use of single bandpass filters in order to illuminate the entire object with light of the same wavelength. This rules out the use of continuous interference filters. On the other hand, tunable liquid crystal filters are now on the market that allow continuous wavelength tuning over the visible spectrum (Cambridge Research & Instrumentation, Boston, MA, USA, www.cri-inc.com). These are electronic filters that can be connected to a computer via an RS-232 interface and are placed underneath the condenser for photometric studies. It is also possible to fit them directly in front of the camera to select emission wavelengths for multifluorescence applications.

In cytometry, bandpass filters are used for:

   (i) absorbance measurements that obey the Lambert–Beer law;
  (ii) excitation of fluorochromes;
 (iii) color images made with monochromatic cameras. For this purpose, narrow bandpass filters are not strictly necessary and broad-band red, blue and green filters (e.g. Wratten filters no. 25, 47B and 58) can be used as well.

Barrier filters. Barrier filters may be made of either gelatin or glass. Long-wave-pass filters transmit only light at wavelengths higher than their cut-off point. Vice versa short-wave-pass filters transmit only light at wavelengths lower than their cut-off point.

In cytometry, barrier filters are used:

   (i) as color filters to increase or decrease specific staining or counterstaining;
  (ii) to block the emission of fluorescent dyes at wavelengths lower than a nominal cut-off point (only long-wave-pass filters).

Opaque geometric targets. Microscopic geometric figures of exact size can be used as reference objects and placed on a glass slide as targets for cytometric calibration. A limited variety of geometrical figures and sizes are now commercially available (Applied Image), but they can also be constructed in the laboratory. In the past, we have tried several methods to obtain opaque objects. Graphite powder, which is commonly used in cytometry to measure glare (Chieco *et al.*, 1994), is of irregular shape, thick and excessively refracting. Furthermore, it is extremely laborious to prepare clean slides with a single object of the desired shape per field. Gold or carbon evaporation through small apertures provides satisfactorily uniform circular discs, but vapor coating reduces the internal hole of the aperture and the technique requires technical experience with sophisticated evaporators.

The following procedure is simple and is modified from Howling and Fitzgerald (1959), to prepare thin opaque circular disc targets on microscopical slides. All steps of the procedure have to be carefully executed using the cleanest equipment and solutions.

Procedure

1. Procure platinum or molybdenum disk apertures (DA) used in electron microscopy or else precision pinholes used in laser and holographic applications.

    DAs should be new or carefully cleaned. A useful series of diameters of the internal hole is 10, 20, 40, 100, 200, 300, 600 and 1000 μm.

2. Dissect rectangular sheets of thin black metal or plastic foil with the size of a microscope slide.

    The foil should be absolutely flat.

3. Using a bench lathe, perforate the foil with holes slightly larger than the external DA width that are at least 0.5 cm apart from each other.

    For a 2 mm DA, the hole should have diameter of 2.1–2.2 mm. The holes can be made in groups of three or four in one foil.

4. Graft a DA into each hole and align its surface with the foil surface.

    A small piece of Parafilm^{TM} (American National Can, Neenah, WI, USA) can be used to fix the DAs in the holes. Do not hit the DA nor use glue. Carefully paint the joint of the inserted DAs and the foil with black enamel using a fine brush in order to fill any gaps due to contact irregularities.

5. Make a contact exposure of the mask with a strip of an extremely high contrast Kodalith Ortho film (Eastman Kodak) in a dark room. Determine proper exposure by using a 15 W light source at a distance of 30–40 cm from the film and exposure times of 0.5–1.0 s. Develop the exposed film for 1–3 min depending on the exposure, fix for 1 min, wash and dry.

Use recently prepared solutions to avoid annoying irregularities in the film. Note that the width of the image increases with length of time of exposure and that low light in combination with longer exposure times provides sharper margins of the disk than strong light and short exposure times. Images of the smallest DAs are usually 1.2–2.0 times wider than the nominal width.

6. Mount dried films on a glass microscope slide with the opaque emulsion side face up towards the coverslip, using a mounting medium.

Circular disks prepared in this way are permanent black targets that last for years. In cytometry, circular reference disks are used for:

(i) determination of glare produced by objectives used for photometric measurements;
(ii) tests of contrast properties of the system;
(iii) control of precision of the formulas used by the software to calculate length of perimeters and curved lines.

Sine patterns. In terms of image sharpness of a video system, the performance is often expressed in TV lines. This specification is an indication of the highest spatial frequency of the system (i.e. the maximum number of parallel horizontal or vertical lines) that can be discerned in an image. Spatial frequency is defined as the number of cycles (i.e. of black-and-white line pairs) per unit distance. Ultra-high resolution glass targets are available that contain submillimeter bar patterns (Applied Image). For video microscopy, it is necessary to use targets with spatial frequencies ranging from 50 line pairs per mm up to 500 or 1000 line pairs per mm. This largely depends on the magnification used.

In cytometry, sine pattern targets are not used frequently because sharpness is checked with microscopical objects such as single cells, cell organelles, chromatin nets and so on. However, a resolution bar target can be useful for comparing the performance of different objectives, cameras, monitors and image compression algorithms.

Fluorescence standards. In epifluorescence microscopy, mercury arc (HBO), xenon arc (XBO), or hybrid mercury/xenon lamps connected to a stabilized power supply are used as light sources to excite fluorochromes. The intensity of these light sources is usually not adjustable, therefore, it has to be checked over time using proper standard specimens. Commonly used fluorescent standards are uranyl glass plates, colored gelatin filters and fluorochrome-charged polymer microspheres (beads).

Not all gelatin filters can be used as fluorescence standards. Under certain conditions, filters fade rapidly. Fading depends mainly on heat produced by irradiation and is therefore a larger problem when using high-power or high-numerical aperture objectives with a short working distance. Gelatin filters may melt when irradiated for too long with light that is absorbed. The intensity of the video signal from filter fluorescence depends on several factors, including:

(i) the gelatin filter absorption and emission characteristics;
(ii) the barrier filter mounted in the microscope;
(iii) the response of the sensor to the emission wavelength;
(iv) presence of infrared blocking filters in the light path;
(v) the integration time set on the sensor.

For these reasons, each gelatin filter has to be tested before it is adopted as a fluorescence standard.

4.1.1 Test for fluorescent intensity and fading of gelatin filters

Procedure
1. Gelatin filters are cut into squares of approximately 2 cm and attached to a clean glass microscope slide. A fine strip of adhesive tape is used all around to attach the filters to the glass and keep them flat.

   With dry objectives, these standards may be used as such without mounting medium or coverslip.

2. Switch on and heat up the fluorescence microscope video system.
3. Switch the acquisition software to live-video and display the modal gray value of the image in real time.
4. Irradiate an edge of the filter to set a correct integration time on the video camera with the use of a $20\times$ or $40\times$ objective.

   If fluorescence is too intense, interpose an appropriate neutral density filter between the emission filter and the sensor.

5. Once integration time has been set, block the light flow to the sensor and record the dark current modal value.
6. Re-open the light flux to the sensor.
7. Move rapidly to a nonirradiated area of the filter and start reading fluorescence as the modal gray level at 0, 30 s, 1 min, 2 min, 10 min and so on.

   Dark current modal value should be checked at least every 5 min, by blocking light to the sensor.

8. Calculate fading by plotting 'gray level – dark current' against 'time'.

   With a low power objective it is possible to observe the area of the filter with the faded fluorescence as a darker spot on the filter.

Not all filters fade. Some filters even increase emission with time during irradiation. For example, this is the case with the Wratten 58 green and 23A red filters that melt when irradiated with blue light.

To compare the intensity of fluorescence of various filters, it is possible to *standardize emission* at, say, 100 ms of integration time using the formula

$$\frac{\dfrac{GL}{T} - DC}{ms} \times 100$$

where GL is the modal gray level of the fluorescent image, T is transmission of the interposed density filter ($T = 1$, when no filter is interposed), DC is the modal gray level of the dark current image, and ms is integration time in the sensor.

Filters that appear to be intensely fluorescent and slow fading are then tested with low power ($2.5–6 \times$) objectives and long-working distance to evaluate whether their brightness and absence of fading at low magnification make them suitable to be adopted as fluorescence standards to periodically check intensity of illumination.

Gelatin filters may be used for image shading correction. This operation requires the collection of uniform fluorescent flat fields. To avoid a differential fading effect between the center and periphery of the field (an unwanted effect that can occur with prolonged irradiation), it is always advisable to collect the flat field during the first 30 s of illumination.

In our laboratory, we tested a series of gelatin filters and selected a few for fluorescence calibration. The Cibachrome-A gelatin filters of the M (magenta), Y (yellow) and C (cyan) series (Ilford, Basildon, UK, www.ilford.com) are fluorescent filters that fade very slowly. Each series consists of six differently pigmented filters that emit a variety of fluorescence intensities. The Kodak Wratten no. 22 filter is dark yellow and is highly fluorescent and hardly fading. It can be used with either fluorescein isothiocyanate (FITC) or tetramethylrhodamine isothiocyanate (TRITC) fluorescence and low- and high-power objectives. The Wratten 47B blue filter (commonly used to collect RGB images) is a highly fluorescent slow-fading filter that may be used at low power for TRITC fluorescence and at mid power ($6–10 \times$) with either FITC or TRITC.

Fluorescent microspheres (or beads) are available with sizes in the range of 0.1–90 µm and are loaded with one, two or three fluorochromes (Beckman Coulter, Fullerton, CA, USA, www.beckmancoulter.com; Molecular Probes, Eugene, OR, USA, www.molecularprobes.com; Polysciences, Warrington, PA, USA, www.polyscience.com). The fluorescence intensity of the microspheres correlates with the cube of their diameter. Microspheres are used in properly diluted suspensions (3–5 µl) that are evenly spread over a clean coverslip with the use of a pipette tip. The coverslip is dried and the beads are mounted in a small drop of distilled water on a clean glass microscope slide. The coverslip edges are sealed with nail polish or something similar to avoid evaporation. Fluorescence intensity is varied by using different microsphere concentrations. Fading of fluorochrome-loaded microspheres has to be determined with the same procedure as is used for gelatin filters.

In cytometry, standards for emission of fluorescence are used for:

(i) monitoring, and compensation for fluctuations over time of intensity of excitation light;
(ii) as a reference to normalize emission of different specimens;
(iii) assessment of nonuniformity of illumination;
(iv) correction of image shifts due to the use of different barrier filters in the reconstruction of multicolored fluorescent images (labeled microspheres only).

Luminescence standards. In luminescence, all emitted light originates from the object since there is no external light source. During luminescence studies, a standard with long-term stability is only needed for calibration and control of the output of the light detecting sensor and for image correction for shading. For these purposes, light-emitting diodes (LED), chemiluminescent microspheres or nylon nets are used.

Stabilized LED sources of various wavelengths with feedback circuits for the selection of light intensity can be positioned in the focal plane of the microscope as described by Beach and Duling (1993). These LEDs are introduced in plastic diffusers to create a uniformly illuminated flat field.

Chemiluminescent microspheres (Polysciences) are 1–10 μm in size, loaded with dyes, such as luminol, and activated by specific reagents, such as peroxidase.

Chemiluminescent microspheres are used to test the entire system performance including reagents and injector function (Berthold *et al.*, 2000) besides checking the light detector. Obviously, microspheres have to be mounted and observed in a buffered liquid environment to allow chemical activation.

Similarly, enzymes that are chemically immobilized on nylon nets may be assembled in the laboratory as described by Roda *et al.* (1996) and are used to test the luminescent system as is done with microspheres.

Position grids. Graphic software can be used to draw simple square grid test systems with varying internal frame sizes (0.5, 1.0, 1.5 mm, etc.). These grids can be impressed on a transparent photographic film using a phototypesetter with a resolution of at least 2500 dpi. Films with grids are then dimensioned and attached to a glass plate larger than a conventional microscope slide. The plate with grids is positioned under the transparent specimen to provide reference points for field selection.

In cytometry, position grids provide reference points to divide histological sections and cytological preparations into a defined number of measuring fields for systematic or random measurements in the absence of a computer-driven motorized table (see Section 3.2.2).

4.2 Alignment of the light source

An essential requirement in image cytometry is uniform illumination of the object and image sensor in order to avoid time-consuming image processing and to guarantee rapid and reliable morphometric and photometric measurements. As far as bright field illumination is concerned, light-alignment mechanisms of modern microscopes are generally adequate for fine adjustments. Alignment mechanisms for epifluorescence illumination are not always optimal.

Procedures follow to align transmitted and incident light correctly.

Procedure

(A) General setup

1. Use acquisition software that is capable of displaying control gray levels of the image (lowest, modal and highest levels) in real time and that allows evaluation of modal gray levels of small frames in the digitized image.

    It is not necessary to read all image pixels to determine the control gray levels. A reading of one every 20 pixels in any third line reduces calculation workload and provides reliable measurements.

2. Once the light source and the camera are switched on, the system has to heat up for a few minutes.

(B) Transmitted light (diascopic illumination)

1. Select a properly clean slide with a stained specimen.
2. Focus the specimen and align for Koehler illumination:

    2.1. Close and center the field diaphragm while keeping the object in focus.
    2.2. Open the field diaphragm as far as just outside the field of vision in the object plane.
    2.3. Keep the aperture diaphragm of the condenser slightly larger than the numerical aperture of the objective.

3. Move to an empty area in the slide.
4. Regulate illumination using live-video settings so that the highest gray level is one or two units lower that the maximum value on the gray scale.

    This regulation will provide a high dynamic range while avoiding 'clipping'. Clipping occurs when excessive illumination causes gray levels to accumulate at the brightest value.

5. Check the gray level histogram, which should peak near the high end of the gray scale and be narrow and symmetric.

When clipping is shown as a tall bar at the very right end of the scale, reduce illumination.

Note that several 8 bit commercial framegrabbers do not allow the use of all 256 gray levels that are available on the gray scale. Clipping may already start when the brightest pixel reads 240. This is not a desirable feature and should not happen in units sold for cytometrical purposes.

6. Check for uniformity of the field by reading the modal value of a small frame at the center and at the edges of the digitized image.

(C) Incident light (episcopic illumination)

1. Mount a proper uniform fluorescence or reflectance standard.
2. Select the same objective and illumination conditions that are used for measurements.
3. Focus and center the epi-field diaphragm on the standard.
4. Open the field diaphragm at the edge of the field of vision.
5. When a fading fluorescent standard is used, move to an unirradiated area.
6. Digitize the field during the first 30 s of irradiation.

   Prolonged irradiation of a fading fluorescent standard may introduce differences in fading between the center and the periphery of the field.

7. Select an area that can be considered to be uniformly illuminated by reading the modal value of a small frame that is moved through the image.

   The lamp should be adjusted to provide the best possible uniform illumination. However, when high pressure arc lamps are used, illumination may not be so uniform as for a bright field illumination.

4.3 Photometric calibration

Video camera sensors can be used as photometric heads to read absorbance values or fluorescence intensities as a measure for a given substance in the examined object. The photometric calibration procedures that follow are optimized for cytometric analysis of objects that have a size of tens or hundreds of pixels. Therefore, final measurements are expressed as modal, mean or sum of pixel values. This approach considerably reduces statistical errors due to pixel-to-pixel or image-to-image variations. Image averaging procedures are usually not necessary.

Procedures follow that describe calibration of video camera output in densitometric, fluorometric, luminometric and reflectance units.

4.3.1 *Setup for all calibrations*

Procedure

1. Select a camera with a monochrome sensor, preferably coupled with a 10 or 12 bit A/D conversion.
2. The automatic gain control (AGC) on the camera or framegrabber has to be switched off.
3. When settings of the video camera are changed, integration time, gain and offset levels have to be recorded.

   All photometric calibrations depend on a set of exposure conditions.

4.3.2 *Thermal stabilization test*

The dark current level of the sensor increases with increasing heat developed by the camera electronics during operation. Although heat production may be controlled by cooling mechanisms, it is a rule to test how long it takes for the camera response and light source to stabilize by reaching a thermal steady state.

Procedure

1. Select an integration time close to that used during cytometric analysis.
2. Set bright field illumination and focus, as described under 'light alignment/transmitted light'.
3. Block the light flux to the video camera.
4. Collect a dark image and read the modal gray value at time 0.
5. Deblock the light flow and read the modal gray value at time 0.
6. At 5, 10, 20, 60, 90 and 120 min block the light flux again, record the modal value of a dark image, deblock the light flux and record the modal value of the image.

   When longer periods of analysis are planned or dark current does not stabilize, extend the measurements.
   It is a rule to check the focusing of the bright image at every measurement interval.

7. When necessary, repeat the measurements with a series of integration times and/or environmental temperatures.
8. Construct graphs of modal gray values of both bright and dark images against time.

   Periods of response stability of the camera can be established on the basis of the graphs.

4.3.3 Dark current test

Dark current levels increase with increasing integration time and this is particularly evident when non-cooled cameras are used. The dark current contribution to the video signal at different integration times has to be tested.

Procedure

1. Set bright field illumination and focus, as described under 'light alignment/transmitted light'.
2. Set $\gamma = 1$ on the video camera.
3. Select a short integration time and a low-level illumination.

    With an 8 bit system start at 20 ms integration time with an illumination intensity that yields a modal gray level of approximately 20.
    Dark current does not depend on wavelength and, therefore, either white or monochromatic light may be used in this test.

4. Read the modal gray level (GL) of the flat field.
5. Block the light flux to the sensor and read the modal GL of the dark image (dark current).
6. Open the light flux to the camera, increase the integration time with intervals of 10 ms, and repeat steps 4 and 5.

    Stop measurements when gray values in the flat field reach the highest gray level available.

6. Regress 'GL$_{\text{flat field}}$ − GL$_{\text{dark}}$' against ms of integration times.

    The equation should fit a linear regression with $R^2 > 0.99$.

4.3.4 Calibration by gray level mapping and test of densitometric linearity

The same procedure is used to test the linearity of the video camera output against transmission (T) or to permanently calibrate gray levels in densitometric units. A LUT is constructed and saved with specific T and/or OD values being assigned to each gray level.

Permanent calibration is mainly adopted for routine work using transmitted light and standard signal video cameras with a fixed short integration time (30–60 ms) and fixed dark current. The main advantages rely on the possibility of storing calibration tables in the memory and using nonlinear γ (e.g. $\gamma = 0.45$) for photometric measurements. A γ set below 1 is especially useful for 8 bit signals because it increases the available gray levels at high densities (Chieco *et al.*, 1994). This calibration is also necessary when the sensor has a logarithmic or otherwise non-linear response to incident light.

Procedure

1. Use a $20 \times$, $25 \times$ or $40 \times$ objective.

    A mid- to high-power objective covers smaller, and therefore, more uniform fields of vision.

2. Select unfiltered (white) illumination or interpose a bandpass filter with transmission in the green region of the spectrum (520–560 nm).

    With conventional solid-state sensors, OD calibration that has been performed with white light or green light can be used for any wavelength between 480 and 630 nm. For precise analysis at higher or lower wavelengths, a specific calibration curve has to be calculated.

3. Set system illumination and focus as described under 'light alignment/transmitted light'.

    The modal gray level of the bright empty image (flat field) is taken as $T = 1$ or $T = 100\%$.

4. Read the modal gray levels of a series of images captured after interposing the following neutral density filters in the light path:

OD filter	T	Gray level
None	1	
0.1	0.79	
0.2*	0.63	
0.4	0.4	
0.6*	0.25	
0.8	0.16	
1*	0.079	
1.2	0.063	
1.4*	0.04	
1.6	0.025	
1.8	0.016	
2*	0.001	

OD filters should be positioned at the level of the field diaphragm. Combinations of filters can be used to increase the number of calibration ODs. In practice, only filters with ODs 0.1, 0.2, 0.4, 0.8 and 1.0 are necessary to cover the entire range of OD 0–2.0.
For a γ set lower than 1, all filters should be used.
For a $\gamma = 1$, only measures marked with "" are necessary for calibration.*

5. Calculate the best fitting linear or polynomial regression curve of gray levels (y axis) against transmission (x axis).

    For $\gamma = 1$, the best fitting regression should be linear with a $R^2 > 0.99$.

6.   Introduce the measured values or the regression curve in the image cytometry software in order to construct a table providing T and OD values for each gray level.

Note. Once gray levels have been calibrated with the use of the above procedure and they are stored in the memory, only flat-field illumination has to be set at the level established for $T = 1$ for each analysis session and each wavelength.

4.3.5 Direct linear calibration

A different photometric calibration approach based on the linear properties of the sensor may also be used. This approach is necessary for conditions in which light is quantified that is emitted by the objects (rather than being absorbed), as occurs in fluorometric, luminometric and reflectance measurements. In this case, gray levels may be used directly as arbitrary units of measurement.

Direct linear calibration does not require the use of gray level calibration tables and, therefore, is also preferred with transmitted light when a camera with a 10 bit or higher A/D conversion is available. Direct linear calibration cannot be used when the sensor has a logarithmic output.

Procedures

(A) Preliminaries

1.   Camera γ is set at 1.
2.   Camera output must be linear as is tested with the 'densitometric linearity test' (see Section 4.3.4).

(B) Direct linear calibration for transmitted light microscopy (diascopic illumination)

1.   Set system illumination and focus as described under 'light alignment/transmitted light'.
2.   Collect a flat-field image with a modal gray level that is one or two units lower than the maximum value on the gray scale.

> *The modal gray level of the bright empty image (flat field) is taken as $T = 1$ or $T = 100\%$.*

3.   Save the flat-field image in memory.
4.   Block light flux to the camera and collect a dark image.
5.   Examine the control gray levels (min, max, modal) of the dark image and the gray level histogram.

> *The gray levels of the image taken with an obscured sensor are, and need to be, higher than 0, as thermal and other noise contribute to the signal. Therefore, the 0 reference is biased*

towards higher values, and dark images are also called bias frames. Bias frame gray levels increase with time of integration because of dark current. The gray level of a pixel in a dark image is the offset value of that pixel.

6. Save the dark image in the memory.
7. Set system illumination as described under 'light alignment/ transmitted light'.
8. For an image I, the correct T of each pixel is calculated by an arithmetic pixel-to-pixel computation of gray levels of the three images (I, flat field, offset) as:

$$T = \frac{GL_I - GL_{offset}}{GL_{flat} - Gl_{offset}}$$

When the result of each calculation is multiplied by a reference GL value (i.e. the modal GL of the flat field), a shadow-corrected image is obtained and displayed.

9. The OD of each pixel is obtained by $\log \dfrac{1}{T}$.

(C) Direct linear calibration for incident light microscopy (episcopic illumination)

Measurements using epi-illumination are usually taken with mono-chromatic cooled scientific cameras at least with a 10 bit depth A/D conversion.

1. Set system illumination and focus as described under 'light alignment/incident light'.
2. Select an appropriate integration time and/or binning scheme on the video camera.

   Mercury and xenon arc lamps are usually powered by a 50 or 60 Hz AC supply. To avoid flicker in the images, an integration time (vertical scan interval) of the video camera has to be selected that is a multiple of the corresponding period (e.g. 20 ms for a frequency of 50 Hz and 16.67 ms for 60 Hz). Actually, it has to be slightly less (e.g. 19 or 49 ms for 50 Hz) to account for time loss in video signal formation. With integra-tion times higher than 80 ms this match is no longer necessary. Flicker does not occur when both illumination and sensor are synchronized with the main supply frequency.

3. Select an appropriate wavelength of excitation or incident light.

   For reflectance measurements, the use of white light is only valid for objects that reflect independently of the wavelength of the incident light. Colored objects require reflectance calibration in different spectral domains with the use of bandpass filters.

4. For fluorescence microscopy, use an appropriate barrier filter to cut off emission wavelengths.
5. Collect and save a black offset image as described under (B).
6. Collect an image of the adopted fluorescence or reflectance standard in the same plane of focus as the object.

> *Focus can be controlled by keeping a sharp image of the incident field diaphragm at the object level.*
>
> *Fluorescence and reflectance lack an equivalent of the Beer–Lambert law that is based on a 100% T reference maximum transmission. Emitted or reflected light is directly proportional to the concentration of the emitting or reflecting substance and depends on the nature of the object and the system used (Jonker et al., 1997b). Therefore, the selected standard is mainly used for shading correction.*
>
> *Emission of the standard should not be very much different from that of the object. The ratio of emission between an object and a standard should reside in the range of 0.1–2.0. When the standard is excessively bright, its emission can be reduced by inserting a neutral density filter between the barrier filter and the sensor.*

7. Save the standard image in the memory

> *When the standard shows irregularities, it is possible to smooth the image with a 3×3 or 5×5 kernel before saving it.*

8. For an image I, the correct emission in arbitrary units (AU) associated with any pixel or group of pixels is calculated using an arithmetic pixel-to-pixel computation using gray levels in the three images (I, standard field, offset) as:

$$AU = \frac{GL_I - GL_{offset}}{GL_{stand} - GL_{offset}}$$

Further standardization of measurements can be made by correcting for the variability in light source intensity that occurs with time. Therefore, it is necessary at the beginning of each measuring session and at regular intervals to digitize an image of the same nonfading standard plate with a low power objective. The modal GL values of these images are then retrieved and stored along with the analytical data to make them comparable to those of other measurement sessions.

(D) Linear calibration using offset and gain adjustment

With nondigital thermionic video cameras, higher sensitivity and sharper contrast for photometric measurements at low light are obtained by increasing the video camera gain and/or offset. This is not necessary with solid-state cameras because a high sensitivity can be obtained by increasing integration time, and offset images can be subtracted by image processing.

However, increased gain or offset could be useful on some occasions, particularly when:

(i) the video camera has a fixed integration time;
(ii) fluorochrome photobleaching requires short integration times;
(iii) very low light (e.g. luminometric) measurements are made.

Adjustment of offset and gain optimizes A/D conversion by using all available gray levels of the operative voltage range (Murray, 1998).

1. Repeat steps 1–5 of the 'direct linear calibration procedure for incident light'.
2. Increase offset while using an emitting standard that mimics the lowest level of illumination (i.e. autofluorescence) of the objects.

    Matching is obtained when there is an insignificant number of pixels with gray level zero in the image.

3. Increase gain while using an emitting standard that mimics the highest level of illumination that can be reached by the objects.

    Matching is obtained when there is an insignificant number of saturated pixels in the image.

4. For analysis, use gray levels as arbitrary units.

    Measurements range linearly from a minimum to a maximum value.

4.3.6 Glare correction

Glare or stray light is a form of noise that arises when photometric measurements are performed on objects surrounded by a larger illuminated area, such as a single cell nucleus isolated in an empty bright field (Goldstein, 1970). Part of the light of the empty field reaches the sensor in the image area of the nucleus, thus erroneously increasing its transmission. This error is particularly serious when the object is dark and the difference in transmission between object and surrounding is high. Glare is not a problem for illuminated small objects in a dark field as it occurs in fluorescence or luminometry.

Glare originates from reflection and scattering on the glass–air surface inside the objective and relay lenses. By and large, glare increases with the complexity of the objective and is reduced by proper lens coating. Every microscope objective and every combination of objectives and relay lenses used for photometric measurements must be tested for glare. Each absorbance measurement of an object in a clearer background must be corrected for glare.

Glare varies with the size of the object relative to the size of the illuminated field. Therefore, the field diaphragm should be closed as much as possible around the object.

When image cytometric programs are used that do not provide correction for glare, only two methods, based on reducing either the illuminated field or the difference in transmission between object and surrounding, may be adopted to minimize glare effects in cytophotometric analysis.

4.3.7 Field diaphragm closed around the object

When the object fills up the image area, the field diaphragm should be closed just around the image area. However, when the object is smaller than the image area (e.g. a cell nucleus) the field diaphragm should be closed around the object, leaving only a small rim of background light around it to prevent vignetting. Before measuring the object, the light intensity in the empty illuminated field should be set for $T = 1$. This procedure is time consuming because every object must be positioned in the center of the image and measured individually.

4.3.8 Objects stained lightly

Another procedure to diminish errors due to glare is to keep the staining intensity of the object as small as possible, commonly below 0.2 OD ($> 0.6\ T$). This is not always possible and creates problems during object segmentation because lightly stained elements are scarcely contrasted.

4.3.9 Software glare correction

A microscope objective may be tested for glare and a glare correction routine may be introduced in an image cytometric program or in a spreadsheet.

4.3.10 Test for glare

Procedure

1. Set the system for photometric measurement (see Section 4.3.4 or 4.3.5).

    The field diaphragm should be closed just outside the image area. For precise determination of glare, it is advisable to use the same wavelength as is used for the actual analysis.

2. Position an opaque circular target disk (see Section 4.1) in the center of the field of view.
3. Measure the object size in pixels or μm.
4. Read T in a central frame of the object.

    Object borders may be affected by loss of contrast and should not be included in the measured frame.
    The T that is read on the opaque nontransmitting disk is a measure of glare in a given setup of objective, relay lenses and size of the illuminated field.

5. Repeat steps 2–4 with a larger disk.

   Commonly used dimensions for the diameter of the two disks are approximately 20 and 80 μm for 40× magnification, 30 and 100 μm for 25× magnification, 100 and 300 μm for 10× magnification.
   Do not use excessively small disks to avoid problems related to loss of contrast and diffraction.

6. Regress the T of the two objects against the log transformed object area (in number of pixels or in μm^2).

   The intercept of the line at x = 0 (log 1) is glare for one pixel or a 1 μm² large object. The amount of glare (G) associated with a given object is obtained from the regression line:

   $$G = intercept - \beta \times object\ area$$

   in which β is the coefficient of regression.

7. Repeat this procedure for every objective or combination of objective and relay lens used for photometric measurement.

4.3.11 Glare correction

Procedure

1. Calculate the IOD, the area of the object and the T of the surrounding field (i.e. transmission of the entire image without object).
2. Derive T of the object from the IOD, using the formula

   $$T_{obj} = 10^{-(IOD/area)}$$

   As we have discussed in relation to distributional error (Section 3.2.1), correct photometric measurements can only be obtained by summing up the ODs of individual pixels of the object. Therefore, it is necessary to calculate the T of the object from its IOD.

3. Calculate maximum glare (G_{max}) associated with the object area with the regression formula obtained with the procedure 'Test for glare' (see Section 4.3.10).

   The G_{max} is the glare that affects the measurement of the object when its surrounding is empty (T_{surr} = 1).

4. Calculate actual glare (G) with the formula: $G_{max} \times T_{surr}$.
5. Calculate corrected T of the object (Goldstein, 1970) with the formula:

   $$T_{corr} = \frac{T_{obj} - G}{1 - G}$$

6. Derive the correct IOD with the formula:

   $$IOD_{corr} = \log \frac{1}{T_{corr}} \times object\ area$$

A spreadsheet table should look like this:

Object no.	IOD	Area	T_{obj}	T_{surr}	G_{max}	G	T_{corr}	OD_{corr}	IOD_{corr}
1	*value*	*value*	$10^{-(IOD/area)}$	*value*	*value*	$G_{max} \times \dfrac{1}{T_{surr}}$	$\dfrac{T_{obj} - G}{1 - G}$	$Log \dfrac{1}{T_{corr}}$	$OD_{corr} \times$ area

4.3.12 *Software accuracy test for photometric measurements*

This test is used to examine whether software correctly transforms gray levels into ODs at the single pixel level.

> *This test has to be done after one of the photometric calibration procedures described above.*
> *To calculate the mean OD of a field, we have to sum up first the ODs of every individual pixel to obtain IOD. The mean OD of the field is then calculated by dividing IOD by the number of pixels in the field. Algorithms to calculate the mean OD from mean gray levels produce wrong and excessively low OD measurements (Altman, 1975; Goldstein, 1971).*

Procedure

1. Set the system for photometric measurements, using a $10 \times$ objective.

    Monochromatic light is not necessary.

2. Collect an image divided into halves: one with transmission close to 100% (OD = 0) and one with transmission close to 1% (OD = 2).

    Mount a small square of a gelatin filter with OD = 2 on a glass microscope slide using mounting medium and coverslip and collect an image of part of the filter and its surrounding.

3. Position a measuring frame in the white area and determine the mean OD (OD_{white}).
4. Position the frame in the dark area and determine the mean OD (OD_{dark}).
5. Position the frame half over the white area and half over the dark area and determine the mean OD of the frame.

The outcome of this measurement should approximate (OD_{white}+ OD_{dark})/2. When the OD value is significantly lower, the measurement is wrong and the algorithms of the software should be checked.

For example, given OD_{white} = 0.01 and OD_{dark} = 1.55, then $OD_{50\%}$ should be close to 1.56/2 = 0.78. Wrong algorithms produce an OD value close to 0.30.

4.4 Planar calibration

4.4.1 Pixel length calibration

Procedures are described to assign length in micrometers to the width and height of pixels in images.

Procedure

1. Set system illumination as described under Section 4.1.1(B).
2. Focus on the scale of a stage micrometer using a 10× objective.
3. Align the scale horizontally in the image by turning the video camera or the microscope stage.
4. Digitize and save an image of 500 μm of the scale.

    The 500 μm length is arbitrary and any other length covering at least three-quarters of the sensor might do as well.

5. Repeat the same operation with the scale aligned vertically and save an image.

    Obviously, a single image is sufficient when a two-axis (x, y) micrometer is used.

6. Import images into the analysis software and retrieve the number of pixels covering the 500 μm length in horizontal and vertical directions.
7. Calculate the length in μm of the two sides of a pixel, H (μm) and V (μm) at ×10 using the formula:

    $$500 \text{ μm/number of pixels}$$

    The pixel area in μm² is also the size of the photometric spot.

8. Calculate the number of pixels per μm in both directions, H (pixels) and V (pixels) using the formula:

    $$\text{number of pixels/500 μm}$$

    The pixel aspect ratio is calculated as $\dfrac{H_{pixels}}{V_{pixels}}$ *or* $\dfrac{V_{\mu m}}{H_{\mu m}}$

9. Construct a table with measurements for all objectives and intermediate optics (relay lenses and tube oculars) combinations:

Objective	Ratio objective/10	Intermediate optics	Pixel size H (μm)	V (μm)	Pixels per μm H (pixels)	V (pixels)
10×	1	1×	H_{10}	V_{10}	Hp_{10}	Vp_{10}
6×	0.6	1×	$H_{10}/0.6$	$V_{10}/0.6$	$Hp_{10} \times 0.6$	$Vp_{10} \times 0.6$
25×	2.5	1×	$H_{10}/2.5$	$V_{10}/2.5$	$Hp_{10} \times 2.5$	$Vp_{10} \times 2.5$
...		...				
10×	1	0.63×	$H_{10}/0.63$	$V_{10}/0.63$	$Hp_{10} \times 0.63$	$Vp_{10} \times 0.63$
25×	2.5	3.2×	$H_{10}/(2.5 \times 3.2)$	$V_{25}/(2.5 \times 3.2)$	$Hp_{10} \times 2.5 \times 3.2$	$Vp_{25} \times 2.5 \times 3.2$
...		...				

10. Follow the software instructions to express pixel size in metric units.

4.4.2 Software accuracy test for planar measurements

A procedure is described to examine correctness of planar calibration and software algorithms for measuring lengths.

Procedure

1. Collect images of the micrometer scale in horizontal, vertical and diagonal directions with a number of objectives.

   Different orientations are obtained by turning the video camera or the microscope stage.

2. Measure segments in all directions and control the correctness of the measurements in microns using image analysis tools.
3. Once the correctness of straight length measurements is established, collect images of circular figure targets of different sizes.
4. Measure H and V diameters of the figures in the digitized image using image analysis tools.
5. Extract and calculate areas and perimeters, using software algorithms.
6. Verify the correctness of the software results with geometrical formulae for areas, circles and ellipses, using the measured diameters.

4.5 Miscellaneous benchmark tests

4.5.1 Spectral response test for color cameras

The spectral response test is used to check how well color cameras and software separate colors in RGB images.

Procedure

1. Set system illumination and focus as described under Section 4.2.1(B).
2. Using an empty field, set the white balance of the color camera.
3. Capture three RGB flat field images with the color camera: one illuminated through a blue monochromatic filter of, for example, 470–480 nm, a second through a green monochromatic filter of, for example, 530–546 nm and a third through a red monochromatic filter of, for example, 630 nm.
4. Block the light and capture a dark RGB image.
5. Import all four images into the analysis software.

6. Read the modal gray levels of the dark image in each of the three RGB channels.
7. Read the gray level histogram of the monochromatic images in each of the three RGB channels.

> *The image captured with green light must generate a signal only in the green channel. In this image, the red and blue channels must generate modal gray levels close to the level of the dark image. The same applies for images collected with blue and red light.*

4.5.2 Chromatic aberration test

The chromatic aberration test checks the chromatic correction of microscope objectives. Objectives must be optically corrected to reproduce objects in focus and in the same position at all wavelengths of the visible spectrum.

Procedure

1. Set system illumination and focus as described under Section 4.2.1(B).
2. When a color camera is used, adjust the white balance over an empty field.
3. Select one objective.
4. Focus the scale of the stage micrometer on the monitor with illumination filtered with a monochromatic green filter.

> *Other objects with high contrast may be used as well. Objectives are designed for optimal image quality when using green light.*

5. Illuminate the object first through a monochromatic blue filter and then through a monochromatic red filter without altering the focus position set with the green light.

> *The object should remain perfectly focused and devoid of lateral chromatic aberration at all three wavelengths.*

6. Repeat the procedure for all objectives.

> *When an objective does not appear well corrected, it could be necessary to inquire with the microscope manufacturer in order to individuate a corrective relay lens for that objective and repeat the test.*

4.5.3 Test for blooming and image lag

A test for blooming checks the efficiency of the sensor mechanisms to drain away excess charges in columns of the chip (see Section 2.1.1). A test for image lag checks the efficiency of the sensor circuitry to remove residual charges between recordings of successive frames.

Procedure

1. Set system illumination and focus as described under Section 4.2.1(B).
2. Select a low-power objective.
3. Select and focus on a 100–200 μm hole with a dark surrounding.

    Alternatively, focus at the object level on the image of the closed field diaphragm through the front lens of the condenser.

4. Observe the image in real time on the monitor using the acquisition software with the gray level histogram or values displayed.
5. Test blooming by increasing the illumination over the clipping threshold and determine how fast the diameter of the hole increases and whether an illuminated tail appears.

    If the draining mechanisms function correctly, the diameter should not increase and a tail should not appear even at strong illumination.

6. Lower the light in order to obtain a regular nonclipped illumination through the hole.
7. Test image lag by selecting a short integration time (< 60 ms) and move the hole quickly around the field in real time.

    Comet tails marking hole movements should not appear on the monitor.
    When the image of the field diaphragm is used as object, move it with the screws used for centering the condenser front lens.

4.5.4 Test for contrast resolution

A small object or a thin line in an image often have less contrast than the actual object, and the representation of bright and dark parts of the image may be less than optimal. To make correct photometric measurements, contrast reproduction of the object must be close to reality (or 100%). As a rule of thumb, the smallest dimension of objects should be at least 10 pixels in size to be reproduced with acceptable contrast. When photometric measurements are made of smaller objects, the loss of contrast of the system (i.e. its modulation transfer function) should be taken into account.

A procedure is described to examine the contrast transfer properties of the video system and to determine the smallest dimension of objects reproduced with a good contrast.

Procedure

1. Set system illumination and focus as described under Section 4.2.1(B).

2. Focus on a glass sine pattern test target with various spatial frequencies.

    Opaque circular disks of various diameter can be used as well.

3. Collect images of the bar patterns or circular disks printed in the target and transfer them into the image analysis program.

4. Generate a gray level profile plot along a one-pixel-wide line that passes through the bar patterns or through the center of the opaque circular disk using the line measuring tool.

    Objects reproduced with acceptable contrast are those which present a flat homogeneous central dark segment covering at least two-thirds of the object width.

References

Altman, F.P. (1975) Quantitation in histochemistry: a review of some commercially available microdensitometers. *Histochem. J.* **7:** 375–395.

Beach, J.M. and Duling, B.R. (1993) A light-emitting diode light standard for photo- and videomicroscopy. *J. Microsc.* **172:** 41–48.

Berthold, F., Herick, K. and Siewe, R.M. (2000) Luminometer design and low light detection. *Meth. Enzymol.* **305:** 62–87.

Chieco, P., Jonker, A., Melchiorri, C., Vanni, G. and Van Noorden, C.J.F. (1994) A user's guide for avoiding errors in absorbance image cytometry: a review with original experimental observations. *Histochem. J.* **26:** 1–19.

Goldstein, D.J. (1970) Aspects of scanning microdensitometry. I. Stray light (glare). *J. Microsc.* **92:** 1–16.

Goldstein, D.J. (1971) Aspects of scanning microdensitometry. II. Spot size, focus and resolution. *J. Microsc.* **93:** 15–42.

Howling, D.H. and Fitzgerald, P.J. (1959) The nature, significance, and evaluation of the Schwarzschild-Villiger (SV) effect in photometric procedures. *J. Biophys. Biochem. Cytol.* **6:** 313–337.

Jonker, A., Geerts, W.J.C., Chieco, P., Moorman, A.F.M., Lamers, W.H. and Van Noorden, C.J.F. (1997a) Basic strategies for valid cytometry using image analysis. *Histochem. J.* **29:** 347–364.

Jonker, A., De Boer, P.A.J., Van den Hoff, M.J.B., Lamers, W.H. and Moorman, A.F.M. (1997b) Towards quantitative in situ hybridization. *J. Histochem. Cytochem.* **45:** 413–423.

Murray, J.M. (1998) Evaluating the performance of fluorescence microscopy. *J. Microsc.* **191:** 128–134.

Roda, A., Pasini, P., Musiani, M., Girotti, S., Baraldini, M., Carrea, G. and Suozzi, A. (1996) Chemiluminescent low-light imaging of biospecific reactions on macro- and microsamples using a video camera-based luminograph. *Anal. Chem.* **68:** 1073–1080.

5 Operative routines

5.1 Utilities

5.1.1 Construction of absorbance spectra

The absorbance spectrum of a dye or a final reaction product (FRP) of a histochemical or cytochemical assay is obtained by variation of the wavelength. Absorbance measurements are made at, say, 10 nm intervals in the visible spectrum. This is possible only with either liquid crystal electronic filters (see Section 4.1), a slit monochromator connected to the microscope or a continuous interference filter.

Particularly when using a continuous interference strip filter, the entire image has to be illuminated at the same wavelength. Strip filters produce monochromatic light only in an area that is 0.5–1 mm wide. Therefore, light coming from a strip filter and projected onto the object has to be monitored only in such a small area.

An alternative method to determine the wavelength at which the dye or FRP has its highest absorbance is to determine an absorbance spectrum in a spectrophotometer. Dyes or FRPs are in general not water-soluble and therefore are kept in suspension in a cuvette, or deposited on a cover slip that is placed in the cuvette holder.

Procedure

1. Use the acquisition software and display control gray levels (lowest, median, highest).
2. Position a uniformly stained object in the center of the image.
3. Select a magnification that allows a uniformly stained area of the object to be segmented.

   When strip filters are used, a uniform wavelength is guaranteed only with a field diaphragm aperture smaller than 2 mm. This small aperture may cause the field diaphragm to be visible in the image. Magnifications of 40 × or higher should be used.

79

4. Set the system for photometric measurements.
5. Select the first wavelength and calculate the mean OD of the selected area of the object.
6. Repeat step 5 with a series of wavelengths in the visible range and in the same area of the object.

> *For every different wavelength, it is necessary to determine the 100% T value in a nearby empty area and to check focus.*

7. When finished, assign a value of 100 to the highest OD and convert the other OD values into percentages of the highest OD.
8. Construct a curve with wavelengths on the x-axis and percentage ODs on the y-axis.

5.1.2 Color images obtained with a monochromatic camera

When using bright field illumination, color images can be obtained inexpensively with the use of a monochromatic camera and red, blue and green Wratten gelatin filters (see Section 4.1). The procedure requires still images and cannot be used to image moving objects.

Procedure

(A) Filter selection

1. Use a red, a blue and a green gelatin or glass filters.

> *In the laboratory of one of us (PC), we use the blue Wratten 47B, red Wratten 25 and green Wratten 58 filters.*

2. Position the blue filter at the field diaphragm level of the microscope.
3. Set system illumination as described under Section 4.2.1(B).
4. Remove the blue filter and position the green filter.
5. Use a proper neutral-density gelatin filter to obtain similar illumination of the sensor with the green filter as with the blue filter.

> *Blue transmission has to be used first, because CCD sensors are not very sensitive to blue light.*

6. Once the OD filter has been selected mount it in the frame along with the green filter.
7. Repeat steps 5 and 6 for the red filter.

> *Similar sensor illumination with all three filters guarantee an optimized color balance. It is much easier to match light transmission by using neutral density filters than by changing light intensity for each colored filter that is interposed.*

(B) RGB image acquisition

1. Position the blue filter at the field diaphragm level and set system illumination as described under Section 4.2.1(B).
2. Alternate red, blue and green filters to acquire three monochromatic images of the same object, one for each RGB component.

   During this operation it may be necessary to finely adjust the focus of each image (see Section 4.5).

3. Use proper software routines for acquisition and analysis to reconstruct the color RGB image.

   Color image reconstruction is very rapid so that with properly automated software the overall acquisition procedure should not require more than 15 s per image.

> Tunable crystal filters and wheel- or slider-mounted RGB filter systems are third-party components that may be mounted somewhere in the tube path of the microscope and synchronized with the standard signal of a monochromatic video camera and acquisition software (see Section 4.1). With these components, full-resolution RGB images can be reconstructed fast enough to allow a reasonable full-color live mode.

5.1.3 Determination of section thickness

Photometric and stereological analysis using image cytometry may require precise estimation of section thickness. Nominal microtome or cryostat settings are far from accurate (Stille and Süss, 1983). Additionally, frozen sections may lose more than 90% of their weight or thickness when water evaporates during flash drying on the slides (Anthony *et al.*, 1984). Thickness may also vary over a section when cells or tissue contain different amounts of water. Thickness measurements require interferometric instrumentation (Anthony *et al.*, 1984; Stille and Süss, 1983) that is not always available; however, a few image cytometric procedures may be used as well.

Procedure based on focusing. Determination of thickness of all types of tissue sections requires objectives with a high numerical aperture and a depth of field that is much smaller than the section thickness to be measured (Lacey, 1989). First, the upper and then the lower faces of the tissue section are focused on the computer monitor and the distance between the focus planes is determined using the scale of the motorized stage or of the fine focusing wheel of the microscope (see manufacturer specifications).

   It is important to know that, for correct photometric measurements, the entire object must be in focus (see Section 2.2.3). Therefore, the objective used for photometric measurements cannot be the same as the one used for determination of section thickness.

Procedure based on section splitting. Determination of the thickness of paraffin sections can only be performed with the section splitting method. It has been described by Gschwendtner and Mairinger (1995). The procedure consists of dividing a section into two parts with a scalpel. One part is then melted in liquid paraffin and included again in a perfectly orthogonal position with the cutting edge facing the cutting plane. The resectioned thin fragment is placed on the slide carrying the other part. In this way, it is possible to determine by planar cytometry the width of the second part of the section to have a measure of its original thickness.

Procedure based on autofluorescence. A linear relationship has been found in some tissues between section thickness and autofluorescence with excitation light of 380 nm (Van de Lest *et al.*, 1995). Therefore, autofluorescence may be of great help in checking uniformity of section thickness in immunofluorescence studies. This method, however, requires a preliminary calibration curve for each tissue used in the experimental setup.

5.1.4 Area determination of entire sections

A large object (e.g. an entire tissue section) may not fit in the field of view even of low-power objectives. To measure its area under the microscope we can profit from the fact that, with Koehler illumination the condenser lens projects a reduced perfectly focused image of the field diaphragm in the plane of the specimen.

Procedure

1. Set system illumination as described under Section 4.2.1(B).
2. Place the glass slide with the section on the field diaphragm, which should be fully open.
3. Select a low power (1–4 ×) objective with the front condenser lens switched up.

    The best objective for this operation is the one producing the largest image of the entire object in the field.

4. Once the working conditions are defined, remove the section and acquire and save a flat field image.

    A flat field that is slightly out of focus is preferred so that irregularities are less evident.

5. Reposition the section in the field diaphragm and acquire an image.
6. Perform shading compensation of the image using the flat-field image.

7. Acquire, compensate and save images of all the sections with the same objective.

8. At the end of the session, place a stage micrometer target on the field diaphragm.

   When the image of the micrometer scale is too small, a larger reference target (e.g. a 5×5 mm transparent reticle or a transparent ruler) may be used.

9. Acquire and save images of the micrometer in the horizontal and vertical direction.

10. Calculate pixel area (see Section 4.4.1).

11. Segment the section profile in each image and calculate the area in mm^2.

Alternatively, the image of large specimens may be acquired using a video system mounted on a stereo microscope and repeat steps 5–12 of the above procedure to calculate areas.

Large objects such as entire bone sections (Jonker *et al.*, 2000) can be imaged for area measurements using a diascopic slide scanner. Densitometric gray level measurements are not possible in images captured with this technique because white light is used instead of monochromatic light. An object glass is placed in a cavity that is milled in a slide frame with the size of the object glass and that in turn is placed in the slide scanner. Color images with high resolution (generally better than 2700 dpi) are acquired using a Photoshop® software (Adobe Systems, Mountainview, CA) plug-in that can be inserted in many image processing programs. Scanned images are automatically spatially calibrated by the plug-in.

5.1.5 Procedures for random selection of measuring fields

Cells and tissue structures are populations of objects that have to be sampled. For small specimens, such as sections of biopsies or small neoplastic foci in tissue sections, we may measure the entire section or all foci present in the section, but for most preparations, either cytological or histological, the first step is to demarcate the area(s) in which to perform measurements. In principle, the entire area of the section or cell preparation should be evaluated for objects, but it saves time to eliminate areas where the objects are absent or the quality of specimen is bad. Simple and transparent criteria are the best to demarcate areas to be measured. However, in these areas, microscopic fields of view (FOV) have to be selected that contain the objects to be measured. FOV selection should be random following the same rules as are used for sample surveys (Gil and Barba, 1994; Howard and Reed,

1998; Snedecor and Cochran, 1990). Selection bias is known to occur in FOV sampling to such an extent that invalid data are produced. Selection bias is mostly due to subjective selection of FOVs, an operation that is known as selection 'at convenience', and it occurs when the operator selects FOVs to be measured based on his/her subjective criteria (Makkink-Nombrado *et al.*, 1995).

A diffuse at-convenience bias occurs in cancer pathology studies where 'hot spots' are selected, that is microareas enriched with immunocytochemically labeled cells or mitotic figures or vessels (Barth *et al.*, 1996). Measurements are then performed in hot spots only or in hot spots and surrounding FOVs. Other than with selection bias, the problem here is that the definition of hot spot is naïve and it is a subjective decision how many hot spot counts are necessary or how wide the hot spot area should be. Although hot spot types of measurements of a single biomarker may be found useful for prognosis, the reproducibility of the measurements by other laboratories and their usefulness for model-based analysis or for statistical inference is seriously compromised.

Selection bias is a serious methodological flaw that, particularly when associated with the widely abused practice of 'at-convenience' cutpoint selection of measurements to distinguish groups of individuals, is one of the major causes for the lack of inter-observer reproducibility and the lack of success of various prognostic biomarkers (Altman *et al.*, 1994; Hilsenbeck *et al.*, 1992; Makkink-Nombrado *et al.*, 1995). A simple fundamental concept in statistical analysis and probability theory dictates that any item (in this case FOVs) of a population has to have the same chance of all the others to be sampled (Snedecor and Cochran, 1990). All sampling criteria that are not based on this principle result in biased estimates. When we measure randomly selected objects, all qualitatively suitable FOVs that have been encountered are sampled and measured. Only then is comparison between different biomarkers, laboratories and techniques reliable.

In image cytometry, as well as in sample surveys, sampling is commonly performed without replacement, thus a field is not measured more than once. Therefore, sampling of FOVs requires assistance to avoid both subjective selection and multiple sampling of the same object. These operations can be performed with the help of either a position grid or a motorized stage (see Section 2.2.4).

FOV selection with a position grid. This procedure is mainly appropriate for a systematic random sampling. Only the first FOV is selected randomly or on the basis of a pre-defined criterion. The next FOVs are selected using a pre-defined sampling interval to cover as much as possible of the measuring area (Fleege *et al.*, 1993). The systematic random sampling procedure uses a regularly spaced position grid that is overlaid on the specimens where objects (cells, structures, etc.) are supposed to be randomly arranged (Fleege *et al.*, 1991). The main purpose of the grid is to guide the observer in positioning FOVs in a nonsubjective manner and to prevent multiple selection of the same FOV.

Procedure

1. Place a position grid on the microscope stage (see Section 4.1), of which the reticles are square fields with sides that are at least one-third longer than the diameter of the FOV of the objective used for measurement.

   The position grid is usually attached on a glass plate larger than a conventional microscope slide.

2. Firmly place the glass slide with the specimen on top of the position grid.
3. Focus the specimen and switch to a low power (1–2.5 ×) objective to make the grid visible through the specimen.

   The lines of the grids are out of focus, but this is not a problem because grids are only used as a reference.

4. Select the first field in a predefined position (for example, the left top square) or in a random manner.

   Random selection requires that the lines in the reticle are numbered. The starting field is then selected using a random number table or a computer random number generator.

5. Switch to the measuring objective and collect the first image.

   The optical axis of high power objectives may not be exactly in line with that of the low-power objective. When this is the case, a reference position in the grid must be selected using the low-power objective that allows to position the optical axis of the high-power objective approximately in the center of the field. The central position guarantees that lines of the reticle do not cause shadows in the image periphery.

6. Switch to the low power objective and move to the next reticle.
7. Repeat steps 5 and 6.

   The sampling schedule along the grid and the number of FOVs sampled depend on the total area of the specimen that needs to be measured to obtain a statistically sound amount of data. All reticle fields may be used, as well as one over two or three, or a different sampling distribution may be chosen (Fleege et al., 1993).

FOV selection with a motorized scanning stage. Truly random sampling is not easily performed with a position grid and requires the use of a software-driven motorized scanning stage. Additionally, the scanning stage may be used to do systematic random sampling and to line up serial sections in order to measure FOVs in similar tissue areas in the series of sections. The latter method is particularly useful when several biomarkers have to be analyzed in particular areas of a tissue. When this is the case, FOVs can be selected in the first section and all other serial sections are aligned using reference matching points so that the FOVs of all other sections are taken in the same area of the specimen (Jonker *et al.*, 1995).

Sampling with a motorized stage must be performed in a software-assisted manner. Indeed, motorized stages are sold with a computer interface and a set of control commands that can be inserted in the image acquisition software to guide movements and retrieve positions. Scanning of an area is straightforward.

Procedure

1. Record in the computer the position, dimension and shape of the specimen.

    This can be done in two ways. First, the user overlays a reference point on the screen and, using a low-power objective, follows in live mode on the monitor the perimeter of the section (or measuring area). Points are memorized at the beginning of a direction change in the section perimeter. When finished, the software reconstructs the section perimeter and area by drawing lines between sequential nearby points. The second method is computationally more demanding and requires image analysis and mapping in the computer memory of the entire field that the motorized stage covers. The user saves a low-power image of the entire measurement area. The software identifies the section in the image and retrieves its position on the stage.

2. Select an objective and enter the dimension of the FOV.

    Usually, height and width are those of the field area covered by the sensor and displayed on the monitor.

3. Subdivide the recorded specimen area using the software into as many FOVs as possible on the basis of the dimensions.
4. Record the *x–y* coordinates of each FOV.
5. Assign a sequential index to the FOV coordinates starting at an arbitrary point in the specimen, for example the top-left corner.
6. Select the scanning procedure and start to collect images.

    For systematic sampling through the entire section, start scanning at the first FOV.
    For systematic random sampling, randomly select the x–y coordinates of the starting FOV and then follow the index from that point onwards.
    For truly random sampling, randomize the FOV indexes first and start scanning at the x–y coordinates corresponding to the first randomized index.

5.2 Photometric methods

5.2.1 *DNA ploidy*

Cell ploidy is determined by quantifying the amount of DNA per nucleus. Intact isolated cells or nuclei have to be used. DNA ploidy is expressed in IOD units which are proportional to the total mass of stained DNA per cell or nucleus. DNA measurements in nuclei in histological sections may be carried out only when nuclei are spherical and of regular size and after extensive validation of mathematical formulas to reconstruct amounts of DNA per intact nucleus and to establish confidence intervals (Mairinger and Gschwendtner, 1996). For neoplastic or other cell types that contain irregularly shaped nuclei, DNA ploidy measurements are valid only when performed on intact nuclei (Chieco and Van Noorden, 1996; Haroske *et al.*, 1997b).

Nuclei should be stained lightly with a Feulgen reaction based on a pararosanilin-based Schiff reagent whose staining mechanisms and specificity are far better understood than those of Schiff-like reagents based on blue thiazin dyes (Chieco and Derenzini, 1999). To assure stoichiometry and minimize glare effects, reaction conditions should be optimized to produce a faint nuclear staining only and a counterstaining must not be used.

Procedure

1. Use a 40–60 × objective.

    Mid–high-power objectives have a proper depth of field to have the entire cell nucleus in focus and these are proper magnifications to guarantee an optimal contrast for all types of nuclei.

2. Set the system for photometric measurements.
3. Close field diaphragm to a slightly larger size than the image size to reduce glare as much as possible.
4. Select monochromatic light using an interference filter of an appropriate wavelength (550–570 nm for pararosanilin-based Schiff reagents and 580–600 nm for thionin-based Schiff-like reagents).
5. Mark a restricted area of the cytological preparation (1–2 mm wide) to perform the entire analysis.

    Small variations in staining intensity may be encountered in different areas of a preparation (Atkin, 1969).

6. Check the flatness of cells or nuclei on the glass slide.

    Measurements of nuclei in large cell aggregates, which are frequently found in, for instance, cytological prostate or mesothelium preparations, should be avoided. Aggregates may not be properly adhering to the glass and nuclei may be exposed from all sides to the dyes during staining. These nuclei are usually darker than flat nuclei which have been exposed to the dyes from one side only (Chieco and Derenzini, 1999).

7. Select and image dark nuclei (usually those of lymphocytes) and measure the mean OD of a few of them.

    If the mean nuclear OD is higher than 0.7, select an off-peak wavelength to decrease absorbance per nucleus (Allison et al., 1981; Fand and Spencer, 1964) and to minimize glare (Chieco et al., 1994).

8. Select a field and start collecting images.

    Move in a raster manner inside the marked area using a step-size of the motorized stage as large as the objective field of view. Random field selection is not necessary because isolated nuclei should be randomly distributed.

9. For each image: calculate mean transmission or mean gray level of the entire image.

    This measurement serves for glare correction (see Section 4.3).

    Segment nuclei and measure their IOD.

    The entire nucleus has to be segmented and measured, including empty spaces inside. All nuclei of good quality should be measured in each image.

    Record the type of each measured cell (control, tumor, binucleated, etc.).

10. Construct a table including a row for every measured cell, as follows:

Cell type	Nuclear area	Mean OD	IOD	T_{image}	IOD glare-corrected

Keep in mind that IODs are sum of pixel ODs. To compare IOD values obtained with different magnifications, the software should calculate mean OD as IOD/number of pixels and then multiply mean OD by nuclear area in μm^2.

11. Prepare DNA ploidy graphs or histograms using custom-made or published algorithms.

    The choice of either the mathematical or graphical procedures to prepare ploidy histograms strongly depends on the specific goal of the analysis: a search for a tumor stemline, a cell-cycle analysis with S-phase determination, a comparison of the DNA contents in different species, and so on. Useful methods for calculations of ploidy classes may be found, among others, in: Auer et al. (1980); Chieco et al. (1991); Haroske et al. (1997a,b).

DNA ploidy alterations, for example in cancer, are detected by comparing DNA values of nuclei with reference standards that are usually, but not necessarily, diploid nuclei of the same organism. These may be found as nuclei already present in the preparation that is analyzed (internal controls) or diploid nuclei isolated from other tissues and added to the preparation (external controls). Staining varies depending on fixation. Therefore, we strongly recommend the use of internal control nuclei as reference standards, such as lymphocytes or fibroblasts which are easily found in most specimens. For unfixed frozen specimens, external control nuclei may be used as well, after being added to the cell suspension before staining (Kiss *et al.*, 1992). The use of lymphocytes or similar cells as reference diploid standards requires a correction factor to adjust for the high chromatin compactness which lowers OD values (Duijndam and Van Duijn, 1975). Therefore, at the start of a new set of experiments, it is advised to optimize fixation, disaggregation and staining methods using control specimens (Schimmelpenning *et al.*, 1990). By comparing IOD values of different diploid cells, such as epithelial cells, fibroblasts or lymphocytes, it is possible to assess the effect of DNA compactness on IOD values and to select an appropriate correction factor.

5.2.2 Enzyme cytochemistry

The purpose of enzyme cytochemistry procedures is to quantify enzyme activities by determination of concentration or mass of a colored or fluorescent final reaction product (FRP) generated by an enzyme that is precipitated in tissue sections or cell preparations.

FRP quantification requires no other photometric setting of the image cytometer as is the case, for example, for DNA measurements. However, different approaches in quantification strategies are needed that depend on whether the analysis is planned for measurement of:

- absolute or relative (e.g. normal *vs.* pathological) amounts of FRP;
- activity in large tissue areas or in subcellular organelles;
- regional differences (metabolic zonation) or heterogeneity of tissues or cells;
- activity along a gradient inside a functional parenchymal unit;
- *in situ* kinetic parameters of the enzyme (V_{max}, K_m);
- initial enzyme reaction rates or endpoint measurements of enzyme reactions.

For a comprehensive review on these topics, see Van Noorden and Butcher (1991) and Van Noorden and Frederiks (1992).

Microscope setting

Procedure

1. Select a proper objective.

    The selected objective should have a proper depth of field to cover the entire section or cell thickness and a proper magnification to assure a good contrast of the measured object.

Use 40–60× objectives for single cells. The dimensions of the area to be measured in tissue sections dictates the selection of the objective. A magnification smaller than 10× may introduce measurement bias caused by distributional error (see Section 3.2.1). As a rule of thumb, the projected pixel size at the specimen should be smaller than or close to the objective resolution calculated as λ (in μm)$/2 \times NA_{objective}$.

2. Set the system for photometric measurements.

   Different magnifications may be used to measure the OD of objects of different size.

3. To reduce glare, close the field diaphragm so that it is slightly larger than the image size.

   Glare correction procedures are not strictly required when tissue sections are used that are far more homogeneously stained than cell preparations.

4. Select monochromatic light using an interference filter of the appropriate wavelength.

   Wavelengths of various FRPs are found in the literature (Van Noorden and Butcher, 1991; Van Noorden and Frederiks, 1992). If not available, an absorption curve should be constructed.

   Sections and cells should not be counterstained: only FRP should be present. Alternatively, formation of FRP is measured in time by capturing images after, say, every 15 seconds of an area in a section or cell preparation while the enzyme reaction proceeds (Jonker et al., 1995; Van Noorden and Butcher, 1991; Van Noorden and Frederiks, 1992). Initial velocities of enzyme reactions can be calculated easily when these series of images in time (galleries) are used for measurements of increasing IOD values due to FRP formation.

   When OD values are higher than 1.2, select an off-peak wavelength at which the absorbance of the FRP is lower (Allison et al., 1981; Fand and Spencer, 1964). However, once a wavelength has been selected, it should be used for all measurements in a given experiment.

   When the FRP consists of two or more components, as is the case for red and blue formazan of nitro blue tetrazolium salt, measurements should be performed at the isobestic wavelength (Butcher, 1978; Van Noorden and Frederiks, 1992), which is the wavelength where the two absorption spectra intersect so that the molar extinction coefficients of the two components are the same.

Absorbance measurements in sections

Procedure

1. Select for analysis a section with the highest quality, without artifacts introduced by sectioning or staining.

    In end-point measurements, at least three subsequent serial sections are required. Sections should be of similar thickness and have a similar staining intensity without artifacts such as tissue cracks or folds that affect measurements.

2. Digitize images of selected objects.
3. Measure OD in objects.

    In enzyme cytochemistry, the FRP is usually found in the cytoplasm and nuclei appear as empty. When object segmentation is performed, a decision has to be made whether or not to include nuclei or intra- or intercellular empty spaces. When the decision is made, it should be used throughout the experiment. When enzyme activity is located in membranes, FRP may partially precipitate around the membrane. In that case, it is difficult to select a standard binarization threshold to segment membranes only: a given threshold may select too much and include also areas that are not membranes. On the other hand, a conservative threshold may exclude faintly stained membranes. It can be useful to binarize the image first using a threshold to cover all structures and then to perform a skeletonization process that reduces the membranes to the width of one pixel. OD is then measured in the portion of the membrane covered by this skeleton (Figure 3.6).
    When areas with widely different protein contents have to be compared, as may happen in the comparison of normal and pathological tissues, a correction factor may be necessary to adjust OD values for the number of cells present in the areas that are measured.

4. When ODs of many objects of the same type (such as portal tracts in liver or glomeruli in kidney) have to be measured in a section, calculate the average OD ± standard deviation (SD).

    This SD is a measure of object heterogeneity in the tissue.

5. Select, digitize and measure the OD of a 100–300 μm-wide reference field in each of the subsequent serial sections.

    The reference fields should be stained homogeneously.

6. Determine the average OD and standard deviation of the reference field.

This SD value is a measure of variability in section thickness. Section thickness is maintained as constant as possible when sections are cut with a motorized cryostat at low but constant speed.

7. When necessary, correct ODs of the FRP measured in the section on the basis of the average value of the reference area, with the formula:

$$OD_{corrected} = \frac{OD_{object} \times mean\ OD_{reference\ area}}{OD_{reference\ area\ section}}$$

8. When necessary, repeat all measurements with sections incubated in control medium in the absence of substrate or in the presence of a selective enzyme inhibitor and subtract the average ODs of the objects in the control section from the average ODs of the objects in the test sections (see Van Noorden and Butcher, 1991; Van Noorden and Frederiks, 1992).

Measuring enzyme reactions in individual cells

Procedure

1. Select a field and start collecting images.

   Move in a raster-like manner inside a marked area with steps as large as the objective field of view.
   Random field selection is not necessary because individual cells in a cell preparation are randomly distributed.

2. For each image: calculate the mean transmission or mean gray level of the entire image.

   This measurement will serve in glare correction.

   Segment each cell in its full size and measure its individual IOD.

   All cells of good morphological quality should be measured in every image. The IOD is proportional to the amount of FRP in the cell and, therefore, the presence of an empty nucleus or irregular FRP distribution pattern is irrelevant.

3. Construct a table including a row for every cell as follows:

Cell type	Magnification	Number of pixels	Area (µm)	Mean OD	IOD	T_{image}	IOD glare-corrected

   Keep in mind that an IOD measurement is a sum of pixel ODs. To match cellular IOD values obtained with different objectives, it is necessary to determine mean OD as IOD/number of pixels and then multiply mean OD with nuclear area in $µm^2$.

4. When necessary, repeat all measurements with cells incubated in control medium in the absence of substrate or in the presence of a selective inhibitor and subtract the average OD of the control cells from the average OD of the tested cells (see Van Noorden and Butcher, 1991; Van Noorden and Frederiks, 1992).

5.2.3 *Cytophotometry of enzyme-labeled affinity cytochemistry (immunocytochemistry and* in situ *hybridization)*

Enzymes may be used as labeling probes for immunocytochemistry and *in situ* hybridization. Once cells and tissue are labeled, procedures to visualize the activity of the enzyme and the image cytometric quantification are the same as those described for enzyme cytochemistry. It is clear that, in order to obtain valid measurements in preparations of cells or tissue sections, incubation times and solutions should be under strict control and standardized as for enzyme cytochemistry.

Caution is necessary in immunocytochemistry and *in situ* hybridization with respect to signal amplification and counterstaining, because these procedures may invalidate the quantitative outcome of experiments.

Different labeling strategies allow signal amplification by increasing the amount and/or the size of the reporter molecules (avidin-biotin, tyramide, etc.; Speel, 1999). All amplification strategies are focused on amplification of weak signals and, consequently, steric hindrance may occur at sites where relatively large numbers of molecules are present to be detected, leading to loss of stoichiometry (Sternberger and Sternberger, 1986). Although it is possible to differentiate cells with different staining intensity, quantification of these differences is completely meaningless. For quantitative purposes, only direct labeling of primary or secondary probes (i.e. antibodies or oligonucleotides) conjugated with a single reporter enzyme molecule or mild amplification procedures such as the peroxidase-anti-peroxidase or alkaline phosphatase-anti-alkaline phosphatase protocols may be used (Champelovier *et al.*, 1991). In all cases, linearity between amounts of a test target (i.e. an antigen) embedded in a solid matrix and the amount of FRP precipitated should be verified (Millar and Williams, 1982). Strong amplification procedures do not allow relative or absolute quantitation of amounts of the target in tissues or cells.

Counterstaining is not welcome in cytophotometry. However, if necessary, measurements in counterstained sections may be performed only at wavelengths at which the counterstain does not absorb light. Hematoxylin is unsuitable as counterstain because it absorbs virtually at every wavelength of the visible spectrum. Specific dyes for DNA or nuclear proteins with a restricted absorbance spectrum not interfering with the specific labeling may be used (*Figure 5.1*).

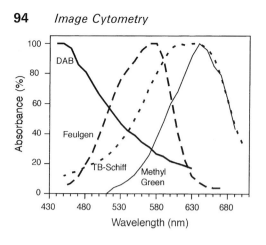

Figure 5.1. Absorbance spectra of diaminobenzidine (DAB) FRP, Methyl Green, and dyes obtained with the Feulgen reaction using a pararosanilin-based Schiff's reagent, or the Feulgen reaction using a Toluidine Blue (TB)-based Schiff's reagent. Nuclear counterstain should be specific with a narrow absorption peak distant from the absorption peak of the specific labeling. Methyl Green and TB–Feulgen counterstain are optimal for DAB-based immunohistochem-ical reactions.

5.2.4 Cytophotometry of histochemical dyes

Several cell or tissue components may be stained stoichiometrically with a specific dye or reaction and measured with image cytometry. A number of dyes that stain cellular and tissue components stoichiometrically are listed in *Table 5.1*.

Once the dye is bound to its target, it should be quantified with monochromatic light, following the same procedure for tissue sections or isolated cells as described under enzyme cytochemistry.

Table 5.1. Dyes for quantitative staining of cell components

Target	Dye	Color index	Peak wavelength[a]
Proteins	Naphthol yellow-S	10316	430–440
	Fast green FCF	42053	620–630
	Dinitrofluorobenzene	—	420
	Coomassie B blue G25	42655	610
Lipids	Oil red O (Sudan IV)	26125	490–510
Glycogen	Pararosanilin	42500	560–570
Acid glycosaminoglycans	Alcian blue	74240	600–620
Reduced glutathione	Mercury orange	—	500–520
RNA	Cuprolinic blue	—	635

[a]Most dyes do not show a sharp absorption peak and small batch-to-batch variations are often observed.

5.3 Quantitative autoradiography

The purpose of autoradiography is to quantify the silver grain density resulting from the exposure of photographic emulsions to radiolabeled molecules introduced into tissues or cells to detect a target compound (Baserga and Malamud, 1969). Autoradiographic measurements are widely adopted today in *in situ* hybridization studies (Jonker *et al.*, 1997; Le

Moine *et al.*, 1994). Calibration of these measurements requires preparation of sensitometric curves which transform density values of autoradiographic films for the isotope used into specific signals of radioactive
equivalents or target concentrations (Baskin and Stahl, 1993; Jonker *et al.*,
1997; Le Moine *et al.*, 1994). The response of photographic emulsions to
radioactive decay is nonlinear both at low and high levels of radioactivity
(Baskin and Stahl, 1993; Swillens *et al.*, 1989). Therefore, measurements
have to be limited to the middle linear range of the polynomial sensitometric curve (Baskin and Stahl, 1993; Lindström and Philipson, 1969).

Density of silver grains is measured either by counting (Lipkin *et al.*,
1974), densitometry (Lindström and Philipson, 1969), reflectance
(Rogers, 1961) and area measurements (Buschmann *et al.*, 1996).
Quantification of silver grains may be performed at low power over
large tissue areas with densitometry or over a few cells or small
structures in tissue sections using counting, reflectance or area
measurements. Two major problems have to be addressed here.

The first is related to the counting method. Silver grains appear either
as tiny single dots at the limits of microscopic resolution or as large
confluent areas that do not allow single grain counting. This problem
can be resolved by measuring the average area of a single dot and then
transforming large confluent areas into grain numbers (Buschmann *et
al.*, 1996). This method is affected by the bias that occurs with image
cytometric measurements of the area of a single tiny grain.

The second problem is related with densitometry and is determined by
the counterstaining that is necessary to identify tissue structures. The
counterstaining interferes with densitometric measurements. This
problem can be overcome either by using reflectance measurements of
grains with incident light over a dark background illumination (Rogers,
1961) or by using bright field densitometry without counterstaining or at
a wavelength where the counterstain is not absorbing (Baskin and
Stahl, 1993; Jonker *et al.*, 1997; Lipkin *et al.*, 1974). For reflectance
measurements a sensitive cooled camera is necessary.

It is obvious that, for a cytometrist, densitometric measurements are
the method of choice for quantifying radioactivity.

Densitometric quantification of silver grains is based on a polynomial standard curve
correlating ODs to specific activities (amounts of silver grains), because the blackening of
photographic emulsions is linearly related to OD units (Piller, 1977). However, silver
grains do not absorb light, but they simply do not transmit light (Jonker *et al.* 1997). Their
density is a matter of area crowding and, therefore, is directly proportional to light
absorption ($1 - $transmission or $1 - T$). In other words, the unit '$1 - T$' is the area fraction
of the field covered by silver grains. ODs are absorbance units correlated to T and $1 - T$ by
a logarithmic function. An increase from 0.3 to 0.9 OD is a 4-fold, not 3-fold difference
(Baskin and Stahl, 1993). Cytometry allows planar measurements, such as areas, and
densitometric measurements, such as T, to be directly performed. A sensitometric curve
may be constructed using $1 - T$ or area units instead of ODs. Indeed, the use of OD always
requires the match with specific activities and may introduce confusion, particularly when
only comparative or relative units among different tissue sites or cells are required.

5.3.1 Collection of images for autoradiography

Procedure

1. Select a proper objective.

    Magnification is dictated only by the field or object to be measured. Low-power objectives may be used for large fields and high-power objectives for single cells, provided that all grains overlying a cell can be observed in focus. When grains lie in two focus levels it is necessary to perform two separate measurements at the two levels (Lipkin et al., 1974).

2. Select a monochromatic or barrier filter so that the counterstain is not visible.

    For reflected light or not counterstained specimens, white light can be used. When nuclear fast red is used as counterstain, the wavelength should be >600 nm, with methyl green <540 nm, with Feulgen-pararosanilin >630 nm, with Feulgen-thiazin <450 nm, and with light hematoxylin >660 nm.
    When the counterstain remains visible, silver grains may be quantified by using a light barrier filter that transmits infrared radiation only (i.e. Wratten Kodak 88 A). In that case, the infrared blocking filter should be removed from the video camera.

3. Close field diaphragm to a slightly larger size than the image size to reduce glare.

4. Set the system for photometric measurements at the selected wavelength.

    When an infrared light or light with an extreme wavelength is used, it is necessary to check the photometric linearity of the video camera and repeat the calibration procedure (see Section 4.3).

5. Acquire and memorize an empty image (flat field).

6. Collect two images of each field: the first filtered (only grains, no counterstain) and the second unfiltered (grains and counterstain visible).

    During this procedure it could be necessary to adjust the focus on the monitor (Lipkin et al., 1974).
    Use neutral density filters to match the light intensity of the two images and avoid continuous adjustments of illumination.
    When an infrared transmitting filter is used to image silver grains, an infrared blocking filter can be used to image the counterstaining.

7. Perform shade compensation of the two images by software using the flat-field image.

8. Segment target cells or tissue sites in the unfiltered image and calculate their area.
9. Move to the filtered image to quantify grain density over the previously segmented objects.
10. For the determination of the specific signal, repeat measurements with matched control sections or cells to subtract nonspecific background counts.

5.3.2 *Quantification of silver grain density*

Measurement of silver grain density can be obtained as detailed in *Table 5.2*.

Table 5.2. Quantification of silver grain density

Software output	Procedure
Pixel number	Precisely segment grains and calculate total grain area
T	Calculate absorption with the formula: $1 - T$
%T	Calculate percentage absorption with the formula: $100 - \%T$
Gray levels (GL)	Calculate absorption with the formula: $1 - T = 1 - (\text{average GL}_{object}/\text{average GL}_{flat\ field})$
OD	Use OD only when a sensitometric calibration curve is available to transform ODs in specific activities. Otherwise calculate absorption with the formula: $1 - T = 1 - 10^{-OD}$

The procedures listed, however, are not always satisfactory, particularly at low labeling densities, for the following reasons:

(i) The output of densitometric measurements is the absorption of the entire frame or object where silver grains are located. It must be absolutely glare-free and the method is not sensitive enough to determine low numbers of silver grains.

(ii) Direct area measurements using segmentation are biased towards larger values, because there is a strong loss of contrast when tiny objects, like single silver grains, are imaged: they appear to be larger and more or less gray instead of small and black.

A procedure can be used to increase sensitivity at low labeling densities that takes advantage of the image cytometry facility to measure both area and transmission. This procedure corrects area measurements using the decrease in absorption occurring when an object loses contrast: the higher the object dimension due to contrast loss, the lower the object absorption.

The rationale behind this approach is the fact that silver grains have a $T = 0$ and the apparent T' that we measure over the grain is due only to glare and loss of contrast.

Procedure

1. Use the filtered shade-compensated image that shows silver grains only.

2. Segment all grains with the binarization tool over a selected object of area A_{object}.
3. Measure the area A'_{silver} (in pixels or μm^2) of the segmented grains.

   This measure is an overestimate of the area of silver grains.

4. Recover the original gray levels of the grains over the segmented area.
5. Measure the apparent T'_{silver} of the segmented grains only.
6. Calculate glare of the objective.

   A glare estimate may be obtained by measuring T over a small very high-density site (it should be at least 10×10 pixels wide) found in any site of the specimen. Glare is objective-dependent and the same measure of glare may be used for all preparations of a given set.

7. Calculate the correct grain density area, A_{silver}, using the formula:

$$A_{silver} = A'_{silver} \times (1 - T'_{silver} + glare)$$

8. Calculate the corrected area fraction with the formula:

$$\text{Area fraction} = \text{Absorption} = (1 - T) = \frac{A_{silver}}{A_{object}}$$

Example
Given: object area = 34 272 pixels; A'_{silver} = 9820 pixels; T'_{silver} = 0.631; glare = 0.12.
Then: A_{silver} = 9820 × (1 − 0.631+0.12) = 4802 pixels; $1 - T$ = area fraction = 4802/34 272 = 0.14.

5.4 Planar measurements and counts

Counts of objects and measurements of their geometrical features are easily performed with image analysis using either segmentation of objects or stereological frames and grids (see Section 3.2.2). Whatever method is used, it is important to realize that objects are three-dimensional, whereas in image cytometry we deal with profiles of objects projected in two dimensions. Until recently, reliable microscopic three-dimensional measurements were mainly performed using stereological tools (Gil and Barba, 1994; Howard and Reed, 1998). However, image analysis enables three-dimensional reconstruction of microscopic structures from stacks of two-dimensional sections using three-dimensional software (Griffini *et al.*, 1996). In addition, three-dimensional microscopic objects, such as the vasculature of an organ or a tumor, may also be reconstructed using a combination of *in vivo* noninvasive scanning and functional imaging techniques such as positron emission tomography, magnetic resonance or axial tomography (Gillies *et al.*, 2000; Strangman, 2000).

Three-dimensional studies in tissue sections are valuable in estimation of the volume of objects and their extent in an organ or tissue, i.e. the number of kidney glomeruli or the length of a capillary network (Gundersen *et al.*, 1988). These calculations are mainly made in the context of stereology and require special estimators, rigorous random sampling, serial and isotropic sectioning, uniform section thickness and correction factors for tissue shrinkage and other potential sources of errors. One of the main topics in stereological measurements is object sampling with a probability that is proportional to their number and not to their size (Gil and Barba, 1994; Howard and Reed, 1998). Instead, the probability for an object to have its profile in a section is proportional to its size and/or height. Therefore, many stereological methods were developed to calculate size-corrected unbiased estimates of the number of objects in a given volume.

Most planar measurements are conducted in sections and cells without three-dimensional extrapolation, despite the fact that they are not efficient as volume determinations. This occurs in pathological, pharmacological and toxicological studies, where either the quantification of modifications does not require three-dimensional extrapolations or a reference volume is not available. Certainly, when variations in total number of objects are investigated, for example, neuron loss with aging, size-corrected stereological counts are mandatory (West, 1993). Independently of the methodological approach, cytometric measurements are performed on two-dimensional images, and this is the topic of this paragraph.

In image cytometry, we sample single objects to estimate a parameter of the entire population of objects. Thus, sampling has to be unbiased with respect to the selection of both the FOVs and the objects in the FOVs. Measuring procedures should be simple and rapid enough to allow measurements of series of objects in a reasonable period of time.

The simplest measurements performed with image cytometry are those morphometric analyses where it is sufficient to interactively segment both target and reference objects in order to estimate areas, for example the determination of the nuclear-cytoplasm area fraction or the measurement of the area occupied by AgNOR proteins in nuclei (Derenzini *et al.*, 1998). In both cases, it is sufficient to measure the area in pixels or μm^2 of the segmented target and reference objects and to determine the ratio of the two data. For very small and opaque objects, such as single or small clusters of AgNOR proteins stained with the silver reaction, it is necessary to take the precautions described in the procedure for single autoradiographic grain quantification (see above).

Several approaches may, conversely, be adopted to determine relative or absolute frequencies of objects in a given structure.

5.4.1 Determination of frequencies

One of the most frequently encountered problems is to estimate the number of objects in a given context. The measurement is then expressed as percentage of reference objects or percentage of a reference area, or as number of objects in a reference area. Measurements of this type are counts of mitotic figures, blood vessel profiles, immunolabeled cells, immunolabeled nuclei, or the measurement of the amount of stroma, nerve fiber density and so on. Two steps are essential: first, the measurement of the target object and, second, the measurement of the reference area or objects. When a systematic or truly random sampling is used, FOVs may be taken at mid and high power (20–$100\times$) because random sampling allows unbiased estimates of population parameters using a limited number of items. This is a great advantage for object recognition. When nonrandom sampling is used, it is necessary to increase the fraction of the specimen measured with either low-power objectives, which may not allow easy object recognition, or a high number of medium–high-power FOVs, which is a time-consuming procedure.

It is not strictly necessary to use the same measuring procedure for objects and reference structures. Indeed, rare objects can simply be counted and reference objects may be estimated using area measurement methods. It would be a waste of time to count thousands of reference objects. Lengthy and frustrating measurements are prone to errors and constrain the observer to measuring only a few FOVs that may not be representative for the specimen. It is good practice to select the most favorable, but unbiased, measurement procedure in terms of time, although it may appear less precise. When unbiased random sampling schemes are used, different types of measurements give comparable results. Measurements can be expressed in several ways: number of objects/ unit tissue area (e.g. vessel profiles/mm^2), number of positive objects/number of reference objects (e.g. labeling index), positive object area/total object area (e.g. labeling index area), number of positive objects/total objects area (e.g. positive cells/mm^2 of total cancer cell area). When necessary, different units of measurement may be compared when proper correction factors are used (i.e. total nuclear area in a FOV divided by the mean nuclear area to obtain the number of nuclear profiles in the FOV).

5.4.2 Counts of objects in a specimen

This method is convenient when only few objects have to be counted or measured.

Procedure

1. Collect a number of FOVs sufficient to cover the reference area.

    The reference area may be the entire section, or sub-zones (i.e. neoplastic foci). It is important here that the entire specimen surface is examined.
    Scanning should be done in a systematic rasterized manner using either a manually or motor-driven stage.

2. Display on the monitor every collected FOV and count all object profiles.

The count may be performed manually using the tallying tool in the image analysis program. Alternatively, properly stained objects may be segmented, identified and counted with the use of the software. This second method is useful when morphometric measurements must be performed in the objects as well. When elongated objects, such as vessels, are counted attention should be paid to avoiding counting multiple profiles of the same object. If this is difficult, a ratio of profile area per reference area should be considered as the best option to express data.

3. Measure the total reference area.

When the specimen does not contain empty spaces, the area of a single FOV may be multiplied by the number of FOVs used. When the specimen contains empty spaces it is necessary to segment and measure the reference area present in each FOV. Alternatively, the area of the entire specimen may be measured as described under the utilities section (Section 5.1.4).

4. Express values as numbers of objects per unit area.

When cells are used as reference, it is necessary to estimate the number of cells per unit area using one of the methods described below.

5.4.3 Counts of objects in sampled fields

This procedure is used when counts are performed in a sub-samples of the specimen.

Procedure

1. Use image analysis software and display the first image on the monitor.

Either color or monochrome images may be used. The only requirement is that objects are easily recognizable.

2. Overlay the image with an unbiased counting frame.

The unbiased counting frame should be provided with inclusion-edges and exclusion-edges (Figure 3.2).

3. Count all target object profiles that are completely within the frame and those that exclusively touch the inclusion edges. Any object touching the exclusion edges or the exclusion extension should be disregarded.

Counts may be done manually using the tallying tool in the image analysis program. Alternatively, when objects are well stained and/or numerous, it may be convenient to segment objects and perform counting with the software. This second method is useful when morphometric measurements must be performed in the objects as well.

4.   Measure the reference area or the reference objects.

When tissue area inside the frame is taken as reference, total measured area is given by the area of the counting frame multiplied by the number of measured FOVs. However, in heterogeneous tissue it could be necessary to segment the reference area in each FOV in order to discard empty spaces and all areas that are not of interest (i.e. stroma or necrosis). Measurements are then expressed as total counts per unit of area.

When two different types of objects, of which one is rare and one is frequently occurring, have to be counted in the same field, counting frames of different sizes may be used in the same field, the large one for rare object profiles (e.g. mitotic figures) and the smaller one for frequently occurring object profiles (e.g. interphase cells). Each count is then associated with the relative frame size and the frequency of the rare objects can be expressed in term of the frequency of the frequently occurring (or total) objects using the formulas:

A_{large}, area in μm^2 of the large frame;

A_{small}, area in μm^2 of the small frame;

C_{rare}, sum of rare object profiles counted in the large frame of all FOVs;

C_{freq}, sum of frequent object profiles counted in the small frame of all FOVs;

N_{rare} (number of rare objects per mm^2 of tissue) = $10^6 * C_{\text{rare}}/(A_{\text{large}}*$ number of FOVs);

N_{freq} (number of frequent objects per mm^2 of tissue) = $10^6 * C_{\text{freq}}/(A_{\text{small}}*$number of FOVs);

ratio, $N_{\text{rare}}/N_{\text{freq}}$ or $N_{\text{rare}}/(N_{\text{rare}}+N_{\text{freq}})$.

5.4.4 Area and area fraction of objects

To estimate the area occupied by objects in an entire section or a culture dish, a few procedures can be used.

Segmentation at low magnification*.* When the object is easily discernible (e.g. specifically stained stroma), one or two images of the section can be collected using a low-power objective. The area of the object and that of the section are then segmented with image analysis software and the number of pixels is transformed into mm^2.

Area fraction with a point grid*.* When the contrast of object(s) does not allow reliable segmentation, a representative number of FOVs may be randomly collected using a mid–high-power objective. The area fraction of the object(s) is estimated using a point grid by counting the points that fall on the object(s) and those that fall on the reference structures. The point density of the grid may vary, depending on the size or frequency of the object(s) (e.g. a 100-point grid for the objects and a 25-point grid for the reference parenchyma).

When the same grid (e.g. a 100-point grid) is used for all counts, the various estimates are calculated as follows:

P_{obj} = sum of points hitting the object in all FOVs;

P_{ref} = sum of points hitting both objects and reference tissue in all FOVs;

P_{sec} = sum of points hitting the section tissue in all FOVs; when the section is taken as reference, then $P_{sec} = P_{ref}$;

A_{sec} = area of the entire section measured in mm^2;

A_{obj} (area in mm^2 of the object in the section) = $A_{sec} \times P_{obj}/P_{sec}$;

A_{ref} (area in mm^2 of reference tissue in the section) = $A_{sec} \times P_{ref}/P_{sec}$;

area fraction of objects over the reference tissue = $A_{obj}/A_{ref} = P_{obj}/P_{ref}$.

When two different grids (e.g. a 100-point grid for the object and a 25-point grid for the reference tissue) are used, the various estimates are calculated as follows:

P_{obj} = sum of points of the 100-point grid hitting the object in all FOVs;

P_{ref} = sum of points of the 25-point grid hitting both objects and reference tissue in all FOVs;

P_{sec}= sum of points of the 25-point grid hitting the section tissue in all FOVs; when the section is taken as reference, then $P_{sec} = P_{ref}$;

A_{sec} = area of the entire tissue section in mm^2;

ratio = ratio of point density in the two grids = 100:25 = 4;

A_{obj} (area in mm^2 of the object in the section) = $A_{sec} \times P_{obj}/(P_{sec} \times ratio)$;

A_{ref} (area in mm^2 of the reference tissue in the section) = $A_{sec} \times P_{ref}/P_{sec}$;

area fraction of objects over reference tissue = $A_{obj}/A_{ref} = P_{obj}/(P_{ref} \times ratio)$.

Area fraction with motorized stage and one-point grid. When a motorized stage is available, the entire specimen or the area of interest can be randomly scanned as described in Section 5.1.5 using a mid–high-power lens. The scanning step can be selected as equal to or smaller than the objective FOV to provide a proper number of FOVs for each specimen. Each FOV is displayed on the monitor and a one-point grid is overlaid on the image. When the point of the grid falls on the object of interest, a positive hit is recorded. The fraction of the object area in the specimen is given by the simple ratio: number of hits/number of examined FOVs. This is multiplied by section area to obtain object area in mm^2. For details of this procedure see Brugghe *et al.* (1997).

Although this last method is quite efficient and unbiased, it does not guarantee precise measurement of area fraction of objects that occur with low frequency ($< 10\%$ of total area of the section). It could, therefore, be advantageous to select objects with the procedure in Section 5.7.2 and measure their area using segmentation procedures in properly stained sections.

5.4.5 Labeling index

The labeling index (LI), that is the percentage of elements that are positive for a given marker over the total population of elements, is used frequently. LI is usually expressed as a percentage and determined in a representative number of FOVs that are collected at mid–high magnification to clearly distinguish cell types. A systematic or truly random sampling scheme of FOVs must be used.

When color images with easily distinguishable labeled cells are available, LI may be estimated using a direct counting procedure (see the procedure in Section 5.4.3). Direct counting, however, can be wearisome and time-consuming when many elements have to be counted. Instead, a 10×10 point or higher grid can be overlaid on the image and the number of points hitting the labeled cells can be related to the number of points hitting all cells. This procedure may be considered as a systematic sampling of randomly distributed objects in the field. The final measurement is a percentage calculated as the number of hits of labeled cells divided by the number of hits of labeled and unlabeled reference cells multiplied by 100. It is expressed as LI area (LIa) because, as is the case with all planar measurements performed with point grids, it is the area of the field covered by cells that is measured.

When small objects (e.g. nuclei) are counted, the probability is high that a point hits the border of the object. It therefore helps to use points shaped as small crosses. A good rule to avoid over-counting is to establish that, in the case of uncertainty, only objects that can be seen in the upper-right corner of the cross are counted. Of course, any other corner may be selected as well.

When monochrome images are used, labeled cells may not be readily recognized. Then, two images are collected. one at a wavelength at which the contrast between positive and negative cells is highest, and a second image of exactly the same FOV at a wavelength at which both positive and negative cells are properly visible. This second image is first cleared of all unwanted disturbing objects and the cells are segmented as black (gray level = 0) over white background (gray level = 255). Once the area of the field covered by the black pixels (i.e. total cell area) has been recorded, the first image is added in such a way that only the black pixels are replaced. An image is thus formed with white background and positive cells clearly visible over the total cell area. At this point, an equalization operation increases the contrast between positive and negative cells. A second segmentation is then performed including only positive cells (*Figure 5.2*). The final measurement is given as area of positive cells as percentage of the total area of cells.

This procedure is mainly used when the labeling is in the nucleus (e.g. nuclear receptors) and requires counterstaining with methyl green or a Schiff-type reaction that is specific for nuclei and disappears when monochromatic light is used for labeled cells. A disadvantage of this procedure is that unwanted nuclei have to be manually erased from the image. If correctly performed, this procedure gives measurements comparable to those obtained using the point-grid method.

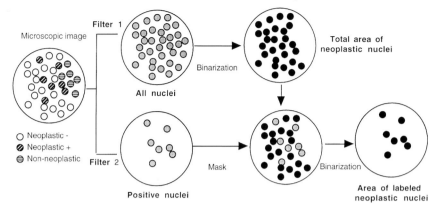

Figure 5.2. Procedure for measuring labeling index using nuclear segmentation. The image taken at the wavelength selected to increase the contrast of labeled nuclei is superimposed over the binary image that contains only segmented reference nuclei. A second binarization makes it easy to segment labeled nuclei only without interference from nonspecific staining.

References

Allison, D.C., Ridolpho, P.F., Rasch, E.M., Rasch, R.W. and Johnson T.S. (1981) Increased accuracy of absorption cytophotometric DNA values by control of stain intensity. *J. Histochem. Cytochem.* **29:** 1219–1228.

Altman, D.G., Lausen, B., Sauerbrei, W. and Schumacher, M. (1994) Dangers of using 'optimal' cutpoints in the evaluation of prognostic factors. *J. Natl. Cancer. Inst.* **86:** 829–835.

Anthony, A., Colurso, G.J. Bocan, T.M.A. and Doebler, J.A. (1984) Interferometric analysis and intrasection and intersection thickness variability associated with cryostat microtomy. *Histochem. J.* **16:** 61–70.

Atkin, N.B. (1969) Perimodal variation of DNA values of normal and malignant cells. *Acta Cytol.* **13:** 270–273.

Auer, G.U., Caspersson, T.O. and Wallgren, A.S. (1980) DNA content and survival in mammary carcinomas. *Anal. Quant. Cytol.* **2:** 161–165.

Barth, P.J., Weingärtner, K., Köhler, H.H. and Bittinger, A. (1996) Assessment of the vascularization in prostatic carcinoma. A morphometric investigation. *Hum. Pathol.* **27:** 1306–1310.

Baserga, R. and Malamud, D. (1969) *Autoradiography. Techniques and Application.* Harper & Raw Publishers, New York, NY.

Baskin, D.G. and Stahl, W.L. (1993) Fundamentals of quantitative autoradiography by computer densitometry for in situ hybridization, with emphasis on ^{33}P. *J. Histochem. Cytochem.* **41:** 1767–1776.

Brugghe, J., Baak, J.P.A., Meijer, G.A., Van Diest, P.J. and Brinkhuis, M. (1997) Rapid and reliable assessment of volume percentage of epithelium in borderline and invasive ovarian tumors. *Anal. Quant. Histol. Cytol.* **20:** 14–20.

Buschmann, M.D., Maurer, A.-M., Berger, E. and Hunziker, E.B. (1996) A method of quantitative autoradiography for the spatial localization of proteoglycan synthesis rates in cartilage. *J. Histochem. Cytochem.* **44:** 423–431.

Butcher, R.G. (1978) The measurement in tissue sections of the two formazans derived from nitroblue tetrazolium in dehydrogenase reactions. *Histochem. J.* **10:** 739–744.

Champelovier, P., Signeurin, D., Christophe, P. and Kolodie, L. (1991) Quantification by image analysis of immunocytochemical reactions: application for determination of lysozyme content in individual smeared cells. *J. Histochem. Cytochem.* **39:** 31–36.

Chieco, P. and Derenzini, M. (1999) The Feulgen reaction 75 years on. *Histochem. Cell. Biol.* 111: 345–358.

Chieco, P. and Van Noorden, C.J.F. (1996) Letter to the Editor. *Mod. Pathol.* **9:** 84–85.

Chieco, P., Melchiorri, C., Lisignoli, G., Marabini, A. and Orlandi, C. (1991) A multifaced DNA ploidy analysis to determine ovarian carcinoma aggressiveness. *Cancer* **67:** 1878–1885.

Chieco, P., Jonker, A., Melchiorri, C., Vanni, G., Van Noorden, C.J.F. (1994) A user's guide for avoiding errors in absorbance image cytometry: a review with original experimental observations. *Histochem. J.* **26:** 1–19.

Derenzini, M., Trerè, D., Pession, A., Montanaro, L., Sirri, V., Ochs, R.L. (1998) Nucleolar function and size in cancer cells. *Am. J. Pathol.* **152:** 1291–1297.

Duijndam, W.A.L. and Van Duijn, P. (1975) The influence of chromatin compactness on the stoichiometry of the Feulgen-Schiff procedure studied in model films. II. Investigations on films containing condensed or swollen chicken erythrocyte nuclei. *J. Histochem. Cytochem.* **23:** 891–900.

Fand, S.B. and Spencer, R.P. (1964) Off-peak absorption measurements in Feulgen cytophotometry. *J. Cell. Biol.* **22:** 515–520.

Fleege, J.C., Van Diest, P.J. and Baak, J.P.A. (1991) Reliability of quantitative pathological assessments, standards, and quality control. In: *Manual of Quantitative Pathology in Cancer Diagnosis and Prognosis* (ed. J.P.A. Baak). Springer, Berlin, Germany, pp. 151–181.

Fleege, J.C., Van Diest, P.J. and Baak, J.P.A. (1993) Systematic random sampling for selective interactive nuclear morphometry in breast cancer sections. Refinement and multiobserver evaluation. *Anal. Quant. Cytol. Histol.* **15:** 281–288.

Gil, J. and Barba, J. (1994) Principles of stereology. Computerized applications to anatomic pathology. In: *Image Analysis. A Primer for Pathologists* (eds A.M. Marchevsky and P.H. Bartels) Raven Press, New York, pp 79–124.

Gillies, R.J., Bhujwalla, Z.M., Evelhoch, J., Garwood, M., Neeman, M., Robinson, S.P., Sotak, C.H. and Van Der Sanden, B. (2000) Applications of magnetic resonance in model systems: tumor biology and physiology. *Neoplasia* **2:** 139–151.

Griffini, P., Smorenburg, S.M., Verbeek, F.J. and Van Noorden, C.J.F. (1996) Three-dimensional reconstruction of colon carcinoma metastases in the liver. *J. Microsc.* **187:** 12–21.

Gschwendtner, A. and Mairinger, T. (1995) How thick is your section? The influence of section thickness on DNA-cytometry on histological sections. *Anal. Cell. Pathol.* **9:** 29–37.

Gundersen, H.J.G., Bendtsen, T.F., Korbo, L., Marcussen, N., Moller, A., Nielsen, K., Nyengaard, J.R., Pakkenberg, B., Sorensen, F.B., Vesterby, A. and West, M. (1998) Some new, simple and efficient stereological methods and their use on pathological research and diagnosis. *Acta. Pathol. Microbiol. Immunol. Scand.* **95:** 379–394.

Haroske, G., Dimmer, V., Meyer, W. and Kunze, K.D. (1997a) DNA histogram interpretation based on statistical approaches. *Anal. Cell. Pathol.* **15:** 157–173.

Haroske, G., Giroud, F., Reith, A. and Böcking, A. (1997b) ESACP consensus report on diagnostic DNA image cytometry. Part I: basic considerations and recommendations for preparation, measurement and interpretation. *Anal. Cell. Pathol.* **17:** 189–200.

Hilsenbeck, S.G., Clark, G.M. and McGuire, W.L. (1992) Why do so many prognostic factors fail to pan out? *Breast Cancer Res. Treatm.* **22:** 197–206.

Howard, C.V. and Reed, M.G. (1998) *Unbiased Stereology.* BIOS Scientific Publishers, Oxford.

Jonker, A., Geerts, W.J.C., Charles, R., Lamers, W.H. and Van Noorden, C.J.F. (1995) Image analysis and image processing as tools to measure initial rates of enzyme reactions in sections: distribution patterns of glutamate dehydrogenase activity in rat liver lobule. *J. Histochem. Cytochem.* **43:** 1027–1034.

Jonker, A., De Boer, P.A.J., Van den Hoff, M.J.B., Lamers, W.H. and Moorman, A.F.M. (1997) Towards quantitative in situ hybridization. *J. Histochem. Cytochem.* **45:** 413–423.

Jonker, A., Tigchelaar, W. and Van Noorden, C.J.F. (2000) Image analysis of undemineralized cryostat sections of bone to study the effects of pressure and particles on bone resorption at the surface of implants. *Proc. R. Microsc. Soc.* **35:** 58.

Kiss, R., Gasperin, P., Verhest, A. and Pasteels, J-L. (1992) Modification of tumor ploidy level via the choice of tissue taken as diploid reference in the digital cell image analysis of Feulgen stained nuclei. *Mod. Pathol.* **5:** 655–660.

Lacey, A.J. (ed.) (1989) *Light Microscopy in Biology. A Practical Approach.* IRL Press, Oxford.

Le Moine, C., Bernard, V. and Bloch, B. (1994) Quantitative *in situ* hybridization using radioactive probes in the study of gene expression in heterocellular systems. In: *Methods in Molecular Biology,* Vol 33: *In situ Hybridization Protocols* (ed. K.H.A. Choo.). Humana Press, Totowa, NJ, pp 301–311.

Lindström, B. and Philipson, B. (1969) Densitometric evaluation of quantitative microradiography. *Histochemie* **17:** 194–200.

Lipkin, L.E., Lemkin, P. and Carman, G. (1974) Automated autoradiographic grain counting in human determined context. *J. Histochem. Cytochem.* **22:** 755–765.

Mairinger, T. and Gschwendtner, A. (1996) Comparison of different mathematical algorithms to correct DNA-histograms obtained by measurements on thin liver tissue sections. *Anal. Cell. Pathol.* **11:** 159–171.

Makkink-Nombrado, S.V., Baak, J.P.A., Schuurmans, L., Theeuwes, J.-W. and Van der Aa, T. (1995) Quantitative immunohistochemistry using the CAS 200/486 image analysis system in invasive breast carcinoma: a reproducibility study. *Anal. Cell. Pathol.* **8:** 227–245.

Millar, D.A. and Williams, E.D. (1982) A step-wedge standard for the quantification of immunoperoxidase techniques. *Histochem. J.* **14:** 609–620.

Piller, H. (1977) *Microscope Photometry.* Springer, Berlin.

Rogers, A.W. (1961) A simple photometric device for the quantitation of silver grains in autoradiographs of tissue sections. *Exp. Cell. Res.* **24:** 228–239.

Schimmelpenning, H., Falkmer, U.G., Hamper, K., Seifert, G. and Auer, G.U. (1990) Variations in Feulgen stainability of epithelial parenchymal cells extracted from paraffin-embedded salivary gland specimens. *Cytometry* **11:** 475–480.

Snedecor, G.W. and Cochran, W.G. (1990) *Statistical Methods.* Iowa State University Press, Ames, IW.

Speel, E.J. (1999) Detection and amplification systems for sensitive, multiple-target DNA and RNA in situ hybridization: looking inside cells with a spectrum of colors. *Histochem. Cell. Biol.* **112:** 89–113.

Sternberger, L.A. and Sternberger, N.H. (1986) The unlabeled antibody method: comparison of peroxidase-antiperoxidase with avidin–biotin complex by a new method of quantification. *J. Histochem. Cytochem.* **34:** 599–605.

Stille, K.J. and Süss, B. (1983) Interference microscopic determination of the section thickness of different paraffin-embededd organ tissues. *Exp. Pathol.* **24:** 213–215.

Strangman, G. (2000) Under doctors' orders for a digital revolution. *Sci. Comp. World* **May–April:** 27–30.

Swillens, S., Cochaux, P. and Lecocq, R. (1989) A pitfall in the computer-aided quantitation of autoradiograms. *TIBS* **14:** 440–441.

Van De Lest, C.H.A., Versteeg, E.M.M., Veerkamp, J.H. and Van Kuppevelt T.H. (1995) Elimination of autofluorescence in immunofluorescence microscopy with digital image processing. *J. Histochem. Cytochem.* **43:** 727–730.

Van Noorden, C.J.F. and Butcher, R.G. (1991) Quantitative enzyme cytochemistry. In: *Histochemistry, Theoretical and Applied,* Vol. 3: *Enzyme Histochemistry,* 4th Edn (eds P.J. Stoward, and A.G.E. Pearse). Churchill Livingstone, Edinburgh, pp. 355–432.

Van Noorden, C.J.F. and Frederiks, W.M. (1992): *Enzyme Histochemistry. A Laboratory Manual of Current Methods.* Microscopy Handbooks, BIOS Scientific Publishers, Oxford.

West, M.J. (1993) New stereological methods for counting neurons. *Neurobiol. Aging* **14:** 275–285.

Appendix

List of practical procedures and tests

5 Operative routines

Index